A WOMAN'S BO

MW01204737

A Woman's Book of Choices

ABORTION

MENSTRUAL EXTRACTION

RU-486

Rebecca Chalker and Carol Downer

ILLUSTRATIONS BY
SUZANN GAGE

FOUR WALLS EIGHT WINDOWS
NEW YORK / LONDON

DEDICATION

TO LORRAINE ROTHMAN
and the other mothers of invention,
past, present and future.

A FOUR WALLS EIGHT WINDOWS FIRST EDITION
Copyright © 1992 by Rebecca Chalker and Carol Downer

First Printing September 1992
All Rights Reserved

LIBRARY OF CONGRESS CATALOGING-IN-PUBLICATION DATA
Chalker, Rebecca.
A woman's book of choices: abortion, menstrual extraction, RU-486
Rebecca Chalker and Carol Downer.—1st ed.
p. cm.
ISBN 0-941423-86-7: $13.95
1. Abortion—Popular works. I. Downer, Carol. II. Title.
RG734. C43 1992
618.8'8—dc20
92-13956
CIP
FOUR WALLS EIGHT WINDOWS
P.O. Box 548, Village Station, New York, NY 10014

Text design by Cindy LaBreacht. Cover design by Martin Moskof.
Printed in the U.S.A.

TABLE OF CONTENTS

A Woman's Book of Choices is the most important book on reproductive rights ever written. Other books will tell you about the history of abortion rights and the struggle to preserve them. This book tells you how to *get* them.

In the debate over abortion rights it is usually assumed that there are only two alternatives: safe, legal abortions or unsafe, illegal abortions. *A Woman's Book of Choices* shows that there is a third alterative: abortions— or at least menstrual extractions—which can be used to terminate pregnancy in the first few weeks.

This alternative should hardly be considered novel or surprising. For millennia, and in every human society, women have sought to control their own reproductivity with the available medical technology. They have used herbal methods, douches and lavages, even pointed sticks and pressure on the uterus. Most such traditional methods of abortion have been highly dangerous, painful, and often ineffective. But they were the only methods available, and often grew out of careful experimentation and study on the part of midwives and other lay healers.

Within the last few decades, though, the development of simple suction techniques has transformed reproductive technology. For perhaps the first time in human history it is possible for a skilled layperson to terminate pregnancies easily, relatively painlessly, and at little risk. Oddly, this possibility has played almost no part in the current debate over abortion. It is still assumed that unless abortions are performed by doctors, they will either be risky, "back-alley" procedures or they will not be performed at all.

But while the debate over abortion has raged in legislatures and on the streets, women have been quietly and painstakingly studying reproductive technology on their own. Many of the methods presented in *A Woman's Book of Choices* grew out of years of research by the women's self-help movement, initiated by Carol Downer and Lorraine Rothman in 1971. In hundreds of groups across the country, laywomen have been learning and developing basic health care techniques for women. They have learned how to examine their own cervixes and monitor changes during the menstrual cycle and pregnancy. They have followed hormonal changes during menopause and developed nutritional and lifestyle approaches to alleviate menopausal symptoms. And they have developed a safe, effective method for terminating unwanted pregnancies: menstrual extraction.

This is not a "do-it-yourself" book. It does not give instructions for performing your own abortion or menstrual extraction. What it does tell us is how other women have gone about doing these things, safely and wisely, through study and group effort. Perhaps that is the most important message of *A Woman's Book of Choices:* that women can control their own reproductivity if they get together and work together.

Nevertheless, this is bound to be an extremely controversial book—not only because it is about abortion, but because it is about women's direct, physical empowerment. There will be efforts to ban *A Woman's Book of Choices*, to intimidate booksellers who carry it, to discredit all that it says.

So buy as many copies as you can afford. Stash some away. Give some to women who cannot afford to buy their own copies. Get together with friends to study and discuss the book in its entirety. Read, think, and plan accordingly. There is power in these pages—more power than any law could give us.

BARBARA EHRENREICH
Syosett, New York

ACKNOWLEDGEMENTS

First of all, we would like to thank our publishers, Daniel Simon and John G.H. Oakes, of Four Walls Eight Windows, for their courage in publishing this book, and for their support throughout the project. Special thanks to Dan, who is also our editor, for his creativity and flexibility, patience and prodding, and for his genuine respect for authors and their work. Special thanks to Assistant Editor Chris Holbrook, for cheerfully and efficiently supervising the manuscript through its production. In addition, we'd like to thank Assistant Editor Abigail Scherer and Editorial Assistant Jessica Green for picking up the pieces when they scattered. Thanks also to Elinor Nauen, for a skillful copyedit under less than ideal conditions, and to Martin Moskof for his excellent cover design. We are both pleased and proud to be associated with Four Walls.

We would like to express our enduring gratitude to Cindy LaBreacht for speed-of-lightning typesetting, her beautiful, accessible design, and for her patience above and beyond the call of duty with myriad last-minute corrections, additions, and changes.

We are greatly indebted to our agent, Sally Cotton Wofford of the Elaine Markson Literary Agency, for her enthusiasm and vision, and for astute matchmaking between publisher and authors. In addition, we'd like to thank Sandra Elkin for the original suggestion that we do a book on menstrual extraction.

We owe special thanks to the women of the Federation of Feminist Women's Health Centers who contributed to this project in many ways, especially for permission to use materials from *When Birth Control Fails*, Chapter 8 of *A New View of a Woman's Body*, and Suzann Gage's illustrations. Thanks especially for the donation of fax machines, underwriting long-distance phone calls, and for swift dispatch of any and all requests for information and assistance. Sisterhood when it counts!

We owe a great debt to members of the Federation's Executive Council, Dido Hasper, Shauna Heckert, Lynne Randall, Lynn Thogersen, Janet Callum, Jude Hanso, Beverly Whipple, Ashley Phillips, and Eileen Schnitger, whose support and comments on the clinical parts of the manuscript, strengthened it substantially. In addition, we would like to thank Vicki Algarin-Randall for her help and support over the years.

We would like to acknowledge the significant contribution of Shauna Heckert, now the Executive Director of the Federation of Feminist Women's Health Centers, who, after long, demanding days, stayed up nights writing "What Practitioners Need to Know About Abortion Complications." Thanks also to Lynn Thogersen, Carrye Ortman, and especially Patti Ambrose, for research and contributions to this excellent and important section.

Suzann Gage's exquisite illustrations are surely the most vibrant and informative that have been done on women's health and anatomy, and we are deeply grateful for her contributions to this project. We would also like to thank Patricia Cronin and Roberta Uhlmann for contributing additional illustrations.

Thanks to Lorraine Rothman, for sharing information about the Del-Em™ with us, as well as for a critical reading of an early version of the manuscript.

We would also like to acknowledge the early contributions of women with whom we worked on *When Birth Control Fails*: Suzann Gage, Marcia Kerwit, Sandra Sullaway-Gibbings, Lorraine Rothman, as well as other feminists who supported the project in a variety of ways.

Special thanks to Carol's assistant, Bob Chatham, for always being there and for tackling every task, no matter how mundane or challenging.

We are especially grateful to several attorneys who reviewed and commented on the manuscript: Ronald J.

Stone, a New York attorney and administrative law judge, whose combination of idealism and skepticism made him the ideal critic; Mark E. Merin, of Dickstein & Merin in Sacramento, California, who has been a sagacious and stalwart advocate of women's clinics in a variety of challenging cases; and Lynn Walker, former Director of Orange County Feminist Women's Health Center, who practices law in Orange County, California, who brought both her expertise in women's health and her legal knowledge to the task.

Thanks to our sisters in the women's health movement for critical help at critical times: Ann Baker, Robin Bennett, Barbara Ehrenreich, Barbara Feldman, Dr. Barbara Herbert, Christel Laine, Cindy Pearson, Lana Clarke Phelan, Barbara Seaman, Stephanie Stevens, and Norma Swenson. We would also like to thank Al Rothman for his help now and over the years.

We would also like to thank Bob Chatham, Gary Karasic, Ken Polotan, and Mark Rauscher for patient advice and technical assistance with our recalcitrant communications system.

We are also indebted to librarians Susan Tew and Beth Frederick of the Alan Guttmacher Institute, and Gloria Roberts of the Planned Parenthood Federation of America, who quickly provided many articles and errant bits of statistical data for us.

Thanks to our families for their love and support: Carolyn Allen, Rebecca's mother, and Fran Mulcahy, her sister; Frank Downer, Carol's husband, and her children Laura Brown, Vicky Brown, Shelby Brown, David Brown, Angela Downer, and Frank Downer, Jr.

Finally, we would like to thank the many women and doctors who shared their expertise, personal experiences, and thoughts about abortion and menstrual extraction with us. Without their openness and commitment, this book would not have been possible.

R.C., C.D.

INTRODUCTION

Worldwide, unwanted pregnancy remains a major cause of preventable illness and death among women. Childbirth continues to be dangerous wherever women lack access to adequate medical care or are not free to decide if, when and how they want to have children. In the United States, women's access to abortion is limited by the same factors that circumscribe women's access to all health care: socio-economic status, age, race or ethnicity, health insurance, and geography.

Ironically, technologic advances in medicine have made first trimester vacuum aspiration abortion safer than tonsillectomy. Abortion remains safe; it is not certain how long it will remain legal.

In reality, women's success in reshaping the circumstances of our reproductive lives has always been rooted in activism and it is in an activist context that this important book should be read. As much as *A Woman's Book of Choices* is a practical discussion of woman-controlled health options, it is also a celebration of women's collective strengths: the capacity to gather together, to nurture one another, to fight, and to invent. It is written by two pioneers in women-controlled health care.

A Woman's Book of Choices is a long-needed consumer's guide to traditional abortion options. It will provide invaluable support for any woman who faces the task of finding a provider to help her terminate an unwanted pregnancy. Downer and Chalker's activism informs the book throughout, making it a particularly thoughtful resource in a period of diminishing abortion availability. Rooted in an empowerment model, the authors assert that women continue to have options, and will continue to have abortions; they clearly describe what resources are available and how to find them.

It is the section on menstrual extraction that is the most exciting part of the book, however, because it makes information about ME available to a wide audience of women. The right to choose abortion as a reproductive option is being whittled away. First poor women, then young women, now possibly most women, will lose the right to choose. Menstrual extraction offers a real alternative which could become available to many women.

Over the years, three major objections have been raised to the use of menstrual extraction. The first and most significant objection has arisen because ME is a procedure that exists outside of the control of medical experts or regulation by the state. It is the implicit autonomy that makes ME suspect to the traditional medical community, and at the same time, makes it important and exciting for women to learn about, discuss, and implement. Precisely because women can practice menstrual extraction free of outside intervention, it has particular importance in this historical moment.

The second concern about menstrual extraction is related to its safety and efficacy. Chalker and Downer present convincing data from their wide-ranging interviews to support its safety to date, and its utility in early termination. Hopefully, more information gathered from more women in many differing circumstances will be possible when there is wider knowledge of the technique.

The third reservation about menstrual extraction concerns possible adverse reactions or untoward outcomes. As described in this book, the procedure is safe; but no procedure can be divorced from the context in which it is employed. Until there exists a system of adequate health care available to all women whenever needed, it is impossible to guarantee that desperate women will not use known methods in an unsafe fashion.

Focusing on the potential limitations of this technique misses the point, however. This book is about choice. *A Woman's Book of Choices* expands the increasing armamentarium of women's reproductive options by detailing the procedure of menstrual extraction, expanding the discussion of access to conventional medicalized abortion, and exploring the potential of RU-486.

Because of the resurgence of conservatism and religious fundamentalism, the subject of abortion touches everyone's life, regardless of age, gender, sexual orientation or ethnicity. It has touched my own family in a profound and positive way. My youngest daughter treasures a picture of herself in a stroller, along with other children of our lesbian mothers' group, at a demonstration to celebrate the 10th anniversary of *Roe v Wade*. My oldest daughter has taken an active part in defending clinics against the assaults of anti-abortion protesters. Each has a sense of her own power and her connectedness to others in the struggle to keep abortion safe and legal.

The needs of my growing daughters mirror those of all women: to have the full range of options to help them explore the complex terrain of sexuality, and relationships, and if they desire it, parenthood. *A Woman's Book of Choices* is an invaluable resource in that quest.

BARBARA HERBERT, M.D.
Mary Ingraham Bunting Institute
Radcliffe College
Cambridge, Massachusetts

Why This Book Is Necessary

WOMEN TODAY are faced with two contradictory facts of life. One is that the United States Supreme Court is but one vote away from overturning *Roe v. Wade*, the historic 1973 decision that legalized abortion. The second is that women have always gotten abortions *by any means necessary*, and will no doubt continue to do so, regardless of cultural standards, religious prohibitions, regressive social movements, or the law. Given this confounding reality, women need to know where they can turn when an unintended pregnancy threatens to impose unreasonable burdens on their bodies or their lives. *A Woman's Book of Choices* was written to help every woman evaluate her options and to provide enough information so that she can make the safest and most appropriate decision, based upon the availability and accessibility of abortion in her own community, and on her personal and financial circumstances.

SUPREME DISASTER

As of 1990, 83% of the counties in the United States do not have an abortion provider, and a shocking 16% of metropolitan areas do not have one either. Even though abortion remains legal in many states, 31% of women have to travel to another county to obtain an abortion, and an additional 6% are forced to travel to another state.[1] Two decades after *Roe v. Wade* made abortion safe

and legal, many women in the United States have already lost access to—and therefore the right to—safe, legal abortion.

As states began liberalizing abortion laws, especially after 1973 when the *Roe v. Wade* decision was handed down, deaths from abortion dropped by an astounding 90%.[2] In the last few years, with the widespread use of early termination suction procedures, abortion deaths have been at an all-time low—about two per 100,000 women, or about eight a year—down from nearly 200 per year in 1965, and most of these deaths are related to the use of general anesthesia, which is unnecessary except in later second trimester abortions.

The unraveling of *Roe* began in 1989 when the Supreme Court allowed a number of restrictions on abortion in *Webster v. Reproductive Health Services*. In July of 1992, the Court backed down from overturning *Roe* outright in *Planned Parenthood of Southeastern Pennsylvania v. Casey*, but allowed restrictions such as parental consent, a 24-hour waiting period, and counseling providing negative information about abortion. These restrictions are intended to deny women access to abortion in certain circumstances. Three key cases that could potentially overturn *Roe* are now winding their way through the courts. The Louisiana case, the next one likely to come before the Court, forbids abortion except when the life of the mother is in danger, or when rape has been reported to authorities within seven days (before preganancy can actually be determined). The Utah law, following close behind, also forbids abortion unless the life of the woman is in grave danger, or the fetus is known to be severely deformed. The Guam law, enacted at the behest of the tiny island's Catholic hierarchy, is the most restrictive of all. It outlaws all abortions except when the life of the woman is in grave danger, and makes giving information about abortion, possessing abortion equipment, or helping a woman have an abortion, a crime.

THE ANTI-ABORTION MINORITY

According to a 1980 Gallup poll, 21% of the people in the United States believed that abortion should be illegal in all circumstances, but when the same question was asked in 1992, the figure dropped by one-third, to 14%.[3] In the same 1990 poll, 82% of people said they believe a woman should have a right to abortion in at least some circumstances. In addition, an ABC poll conducted in 1990 found, by a margin of two to one, that Americans are opposed to their state legislatures passing new restrictions on abortion.[4] Clearly, a United States Supreme Court that does not endorse women's right to abortion is out of step with the times.

ABORTIONS WILL CONTINUE TO BE DONE

Regardless of the outcome of future Supreme Court decisions, abortions will continue to be done. Even in the worst-case scenario, abortion is likely to remain legal in at least 15 states: Clinics that specialize in abortion care will continue to operate, hospitals will do more out-patient procedures, and many doctors will do more abortions in their private practices. In states where abortion is legal but widely inaccessible, and even in states where the procedure is legally prohibited, many abortions will be done for "therapeutic" reasons, i.e., in cases of rape or incest, or where a doctor judges that the physical or mental health of a pregnant woman is at risk. In addition, sympathetic doctors will quietly do diagnostic procedures, such as endometrial biopsies, in which the uterus is emptied in exactly the same fashion as in an abortion. And many doctors who do not do abortions themselves will refer their patients to reliable practitioners who are willing to do them.

INFORMATION NETWORKS

To help women get safe abortions, the National Abortion Federation (NAF) maintains a list of doctors and clinics in both the United States and Canada. A nationwide network of women's groups and active pro-choice organizations is evolving which will provide a wealth of information on how and where to get safe abortions. Many feminist health projects, university women's centers, and community pro-choice coalitions will also provide direct abortion referrals in their own communities, and a number of well-established feminist groups will continue to operate abortion clinics. Other groups, such as the newly formed Overground Railroad, will offer information on transportation or housing, while others will provide funding or loans to help young and poor women get abortions. In addition, a host of national organizations that promote abortion rights, such as The National Abortion Rights Action League, and feminist organizations such as the National Organization for Women, the Fund for a Feminist Majority, and the National Women's Health Network, have large mailing lists and will keep their members—and the media—informed of new legislative initiatives in the battle to keep abortion safe and legal. Chapter 2, "Information Networks," contains lists of these organizations, including their addresses and phone numbers for easy reference.

IF YOU NEED AN ABORTION

If you find yourself pregnant and don't want to be, and don't know where to turn, *don't panic*. In spite of the legal and ideological assault on women's reproductive rights, abortion is not stigmatized in the way it was 20 years ago. Women know much more than they did in pre-*Roe* days, and many are far more assertive about their personal and medical needs than they used to be. Today, a majority of people in the United States believe that women have a right to make sensible choices about their fertility, and it is common knowledge that pregnancies can be safely terminated in two to three hours in a clinic. There is simply no way the anti-abortion movement, state legislatures, and the Supreme Court can put the toothpaste back into the tube.

CHAPTER ONE

Finding An Abortion Provider

THERE ARE approximately a million and a half abortions performed in the United States each year, and 90% of them are done in the first trimester (12 weeks). Of all abortions, both first and second trimester, 90% are done in clinics that specialize in abortion care, while the other 10% are done in doctors' offices and hospitals.

Abortion is not an inherently difficult procedure—experience has shown that even lay people can learn to do it safely—but the more experience a practitioner has, the safer the procedure is. Therefore, most abortion experts believe that if you have a choice between a clinic that specializes in abortion, and a doctor who does an occasional office or hospital procedure, the clinic abortion is your best bet.

TYPES OF ABORTION PROVIDERS

Abortion providers fall into several categories:

➡ chains of profit-making clinics that may have numerous branches in several states;

➡ associations of non-profit clinics such as Planned Parenthood;

➡ small independent providers, including clinics owned by doctors, and clinics owned and run by women;

➡ individual doctors who may do abortions in their offices or in hospitals;

➡ hospitals that have special abortion clinics or which provide abortion training as part of Ob-Gyn residency programs.

CHOOSING THE BEST ABORTION PROVIDER

For women in metropolitan areas in states where abortion is still legal, finding an abortion provider is almost as easy as thumbing through the Yellow Pages. Competing clinics place lavish advertisements offering the "friendliest", most "caring," "comprehensive," or "affordable" abortion service. The primary concern of most women is to find the most caring, competent and respectful abortion care available—it does exist, and many women think it is worth looking for if they have several places to choose from.

In perusing the Yellow Pages, it's best to look under *"Abortion Services"* or *"Clinics."* Skip *"Abortion Alternatives Information,"* which is the designated category for fake clinics run by anti-abortion groups. (See page 10 for information on fake clinics.) If there are no abortion clinics listed in the Yellow Pages, you might try calling two or three gynecologists in your area to see if they do office abortions, or if not, if they know a gynecologist who does. Many communities have medical referral services that list doctors by specialty and the services they perform. Look under *"Physicians & Surgeons' Information & Referral Services"* in the Yellow Pages. Some doctors will willingly do an abortion. Others may be reluctant, but may be more inclined to do one if they have a reason. (See Finding a Sympathetic Doctor to Do an Abortion" on page 34.)

If there is no visible abortion provider in your town, the most direct way to get a safe, legal abortion is to find the nearest doctor or clinic that specializes in abortion care. This can be done by calling the NAF Hotline (discussed in the next section), checking the lists of Women's Health Projects and Womens' Rights organizations in Chapter 2, or going to the library and checking the Yellow Pages from the nearest large city.

When you call any clinic or doctor's office, the first thing to find out is what their limit on pregnancy termination is, i.e., to what week of pregnancy do they do abortions? Many clinics only do abortions to 12 or 13 weeks from your last period, but will refer you to another clinic or hospital that does second trimester procedures. The legal limit on abortion in most states is between 20 and 24 weeks, but there are only 85 clinics in the country (and one in Puerto Rico) that do abortions after 20 weeks. However, if you are 20 to 24 weeks pregnant and want an abortion, *you can probably get one*—if you are persistent and if you can get the money together. (See page 62 for a list of organizations that provide loans or direct funding for women who cannot pay for an abortion).

The logical first step is to have a pregnancy test at a clinic, hospital or doctor's office to find out how far pregnant you really are. If there is a possibility that you are in the second trimester, you may be required to have a sonogram, a picture of the interior of the uterus that utilizes high-frequency sound waves rather than radiation, which can determine pretty accurately how far pregnant you are. Some women may be reluctant to have this test, fearing they may be too far along, but *you may be required to have one by the clinic that does your abortion,* so avoiding a sonogram accomplishes nothing and may waste valuable time (see page 75 for more detailed information on sonograms).

THE NAF HOTLINE

The National Abortion Federation (NAF) is a private organization of doctors, nurses, counselors, and clinic administrators whose goal is to assure that women have access to safe, legal abortions. NAF provides educational materials on abortion, offers training in all aspects of abortion care, certifies abortion clinics and individual doctors who meet a certain standard of care, and provides accurate information on abortion to the media and policy-makers. NAF also runs a toll-free Hotline that operates Monday through Friday from 9:30 to 5:30 p.m. Sympathetic, knowledgeable counselors will answer questions about abortion and provide direct referrals to the nearest clinics or doctors who are NAF members, and will send you a free packet of information describing safe abortion services.

NATIONAL ABORTION FEDERATION
1434 U St., N.W.
Washington, DC 20009
(800) 772-9100 (U.S.)
(800) 424-2280 (Canada)
(202) 667-5881 (Wash. DC residents
and for general information)

FAKE ABORTION CLINICS

By its own estimate, the anti-abortion movement operates some 3,500 fake "clinics," "crisis counseling services", "problem pregnancy advice centers," and phony abortion information services in the United States. Most of these groups are associated with the Pierson Foundation, a Catholic anti-abortion funding organization, or with the Christian Action Council, a fundamentalist umbrella group that sponsors many anti-abortion activities.

"Many of these facilities operate in smaller towns where there is no abortion provider," says Charlotte Taft, Executive Director of the Routh Street Clinic in Dallas, Texas. "They prey on the most vulnerable—young, poor, and immigrant women." Taft points out that many women end up at fake clinics because those may be the only place in town where free pregnancy tests are available.

The tactics of these fake clinics can be subtle or ruthless. Some take a lot of personal information from women, and may later harass them by making phone calls or visits to their homes. Another strategy these groups have used with some success is to make phony appointments for a woman whose pregnancy is advanced, and then reschedule or cancel the appointment several times, hoping to delay her until it is too late to get an abortion at facilities in the area.

"One of the most skillful ploys of these places is the insidious mix of truth and falsehood," Taft points out. "For example, one group in Dallas tells women that their uteruses will be scraped with a knife." (The "knife" is really a curette, a sharp metal instrument used to scrape out the lining of the uterus. Curettes are seldom necessary in first trimester abortions.) Taft says she has seen women who have previously been to anti-abortion counseling sessions burst into tears of relief after an abortion because they had been led to believe that their lives were in danger.

In some states, fake clinics and related facilities are required to list themselves as "Abortion Alternatives" in the Yellow Pages, but in many states, they may also be listed under "Clinics" or "Birth Control Information." In some states, facilities are not allowed to bill themselves as clinics unless they provide some kind of laboratory services, so many offer free pregnancy tests to circumvent this regulation. **The surest way to identify a fake clinic is to ask if abortions are actually done on the premises.** If the answer is unclear, or "no," you might do well to look further.

Many of these phony clinics and counseling services violate state regulations on false advertising and can be reported to the state Attorney General, the city attorney's office, state health department, or the Better Business Bureau. Many fake clinics have been closed down or forced to advertise their purpose more clearly because of complaints by women and pro-choice groups.

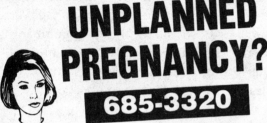
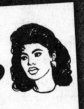
THESE INVITING, REASSURING ADVERTISEMENTS are for fake clinics and "problem pregnancy advice centers," run by anti-abortion groups, which disseminate misinformation about abortion and often try to dissuade, or may actually try to prevent, women from getting abortions. In some states, ads for these facilities are required to include wording such as "non-medical facility," but that notation is often in tiny type and buried at the bottom of the ad. Others offer free pregnancy tests, while others claim to provide accurate information about abortion, but give only a negative picture.

THE COST OF AN ABORTION

The price of an abortion varies according to how many weeks pregnant you are, whether you have local or general anesthesia, and whether the abortion is done in a clinic, doctor's office, or hospital. The cost of a first-trimester abortion in a clinic or doctor's office ranges from $225 to $300; between 13 and 16 weeks it ranges from $300 to $450, and increases about $100 for each succeeding week[1]. In a hospital, an early termination abortion can cost up to $750 or more, and a second trimester procedure up to $2,000.

Clinics often charge a different rate for women who have Medicaid, those who have private insurance, and those who pay cash. Some clinics may have a sliding scale for low-income women, so be sure to ask if you don't have insurance. Some clinics also have a staff person who can help you determine if you are eligible for Medicaid, and tell you how to apply.

If you have private insurance, you may be pressured into getting tests you don't need, or having general anesthesia for an early abortion, because the clinic can then bill your insurance carrier top dollar for these items. To avoid unnecessary tests, always ask if there is a *medical reason* for any additional procedure.

It is your right to know about all charges, so don't be shy about asking. Extra charges may include:

➡ a blood pregnancy test, called Beta HCG, which detects the pregnancy hormone *(human chorionic gonadotropin)* in the blood stream. This test is much more expensive than the standard urine test, and is effective sooner, about 10 days after conception, but it takes several days to get the results.

➡️ a sonogram, a sound wave image of the interior of the uterus (see page 75).

➡️ general anesthesia, which is unnecessary for first trimester abortions, or second trimester abortions up to about 18 weeks (see page 79).

➡️ Rho-gam if you have RH-negative blood (see page 92).

➡️ laminaria, small sticks of compressed seaweed which expand over several hours or overnight to dilate the cervix more gently than metal dilators. Laminaria is routinely used in second trimester abortions (see pages 83 and 91).

➡️ a follow-up visit after the abortion, which is suggested for all women but may not actually be necessary unless something unusual occurs (see page 93 for normal post-abortion experiences).

There is generally no extra charge for medications such as antibiotics, analgesics (pain medication) or methergine, a drug that helps the uterus to contract.

WHY ABORTION PRICES ARE SO LOW

Between 1983 and 1986, the cost of an early abortion increased only 7%, while the cost of other types of health care has tripled.[2] **The cost of abortions has been kept artificially low for a number of reasons:**

➡️ Many clinics that specialize in abortion have a commitment to keep abortion affordable.

➡️ Medicaid reimbursement for abortion has not risen at all in the last decade.

➡️ Clinic associations, such as Planned Parenthood, have low group insurance rates and large fund-raising campaigns; its clinics can, therefore, afford to charge reduced rates for abortions.

➡️ Abortion clinics tend to be clustered in metropolitan areas, and often find themselves locked into competition with each other.

➡Women tend to do comparison shopping, and often base their choice solely on the lowest price.

TO WOMEN getting abortions, this artificially low price may seem like an advantage, but in the long run it has had a profoundly negative impact on small independent providers, whose profit margin is so small that many are in imminent danger of closing. These independent clinics, which may offer the only second trimester abortions in their areas, do not have the economic advantages of large chains, or the fund-raising capabilities of Planned Parenthood. Yet large chains and institutions tend to provide only first trimester abortions, and have policies that screen out women with risk factors such as drug use or specific medical problems. The potential outcome of price-cutting by large chains and Planned Parenthood clinics may be that independent clinics will be put out of business, and the impact on abortion availability, especially of second trimester abortions, could be as detrimental as anti-abortion legislation has already been. Reasonable price increases would allow a variety of providers to remain in business and offer women a wider range of choices.

MEDICAID PAYMENT FOR ABORTIONS

In 1977 Congress enacted the so-called Hyde amendment (named after the bill's sponsor, Senator Henry Hyde of Illinois), restricting Medicaid payment for abortions to cases in which the life of the mother is in danger. In response to this legislation, which is widely seen as discriminating against poor women, a number of states have continued to provide Medicaid payment under certain circumstances, such as if the pregnancy is the result of rape or incest, or if the fetus is deformed. Thirteen states have continued to provide Medicaid for abortions in most cir-

CIRCUMSTANCES IN WHICH MEDICAID FUNDS ABORTION, BY STATE

STATE	PREGNANCY ENDANGERS WOMAN'S LIFE	PREGNANCY RESULTED FROM RAPE OR INCEST	FETUS HAS SERIOUS DEFECTS	ALL OR MOST CIRCUM-STANCES
Alabama	✔			
Alaska	✔	✔	✔	✔
Arizona	✔			
Arkansas	✔			
California[1]	✔	✔	✔	✔
Colorado	✔			
Connecticut[1]	✔	✔	✔	✔
Delaware	✔			
Dist. of Columbia	✔			
Florida	✔			
Georgia	✔			
Hawaii	✔	✔	✔	✔
Idaho	✔			
Illinois	✔			
Indiana	✔			
Iowa	✔	✔	✔	
Kansas	✔			
Kentucky	✔			
Louisiana	✔			
Maine	✔			
Maryland	✔	✔	✔	
Massachusetts[1]	✔	✔	✔	✔
Michigan	✔			
Minnesota	✔	✔		
Mississippi	✔			
Missouri	✔			
Montana	✔			
Nebraska	✔			

STATE	PREGNANCY ENDANGERS WOMAN'S LIFE	PREGNANCY RESULTED FROM RAPE OR INCEST	FETUS HAS SERIOUS DEFECTS	ALL OR MOST CIRCUM-STANCES
Nevada	✔			
New Hampshire	✔			
New Jersey[1]	✔	✔	✔	✔
New Mexico	✔			
New York	✔	✔	✔	✔
North Carolina	✔	✔	✔	✔
North Dakota	✔			
Ohio	✔			
Oklahoma	✔			
Oregon	✔	✔	✔	✔
Pennsylvania	✔	✔		
Rhode Island	✔			
South Carolina	✔			
South Dakota	✔			
Tennessee	✔			
Texas	✔			
Utah	✔			
Vermont[1]	✔	✔	✔	✔
Virginia	✔	✔	✔	
Washington	✔	✔	✔	✔
West Virginia	✔	✔	✔	✔
Wisconsin	✔	✔		
Wyoming	✔	✔		

[1] paying pursuant to court order

This information is accurate as of September 1990. Please contact the National Abortion Federation at (202) 667-5881 for the most up-to-date information. Source: *The Alan Guttmacher Institute, The American Civil Liberties Union Reproductive Freedom Project.*

cumstances. The chart on pages 16 and 17 provides an overview of each state's general policies. These regulations may be interpreted differently in different communities, however, so you may want to make specific inquiries about policies in your area.

The Women's Health Education Project (WHEP) 1992 publication, *Abortion: A New York City Resource Guide*,[3] offers some helpful information for undocumented women who make use of Medicaid funding for abortions. The WHEP *Guide* notes that according to Immigration and Naturalization Service (INS) regulations, undocumented women are not required to present a Social Security card or other residency documentation in order to qualify for Medicaid abortions (or for pregnancy coverage for that matter). Nevertheless, immigration officials have been known to disqualify women for residency papers if it is discovered that they have previously applied for funding for an abortion. However, according to INS regulations, these officials should not have access to Medicaid records, nor should they force women to admit to having had a Medicaid-funded abortion. To be safe, the WHEP *Abortion Guide* suggests that you try to avoid using Medicaid funds for an abortion if you intend to apply for residency status; if immigration officials ask you to sign a waiver releasing your Medicaid records to them you are well within your rights to refuse.

PARENTAL CONSENT OR NOTIFICATION

The requirement in some states that young women notify one or both of their parents before getting an abortion, known as *parental consent* or *parental notification*, has been one of the most successful tactics of the anti-abortion movement. In Minnesota, for example, after institution of *one parent notification*, the birth rate for 15- to 17-year-olds rose 38%.[4] Certain states require *consent* of either one or both parents, while others require *notification* of either one or both parents. In some states, one or both parents must accompany their child to the clinic, but in others, only a note, from one or both parents, signed before a notary public, is required.

These laws, under the guise of "protecting" immature young women and enhancing parents' interest in their children's welfare, have instead caused enormous hardship and pain for parents and daughters. While the meaning of *consent* is somewhat different from *notification*, legal experts have found that if a teenager has to inform one or both parents that she is pregnant and contemplating an abortion, she is essentially being forced to ask their permission.

Over half of all teenagers do tell their parents that they are pregnant,[5] and many are rewarded with emotional support and financial assistance. However, about 25% of young women, afraid of disappointing or hurting their parents or guardians, fear notification, while others, especially those from violence-prone or dysfunctional families, may fear for their own safety.[6] In cases where the pregnancy is the result of sexual abuse, parental notification may place young women in extreme jeopardy. The reality of this situation was dramatized by a case in Fruitland, Idaho, in which 13-year-old Spring Adams, impregnated by her father, was shot to death in her bed by him after he found out about her plans to get an abortion.[7]

As a compromise to pro-choice advocates, state legislatures have provided a mechanism called *judicial bypass*, whereby a young woman who feels that she can't confide in her parents can apply to a court for approval to obtain an abortion. But in almost every case, judicial bypass is a nightmare for young women, and sometimes for their parents as well.

A survey done by the Alan Guttmacher Institute[8] reveals that nearly 10% of young women who are forced to choose between parental notification and judicial bypass, say they would choose neither—that they would attempt to self-abort, or would try to obtain an illegal abortion. In a widely publicized Indiana case, Becky Bell, a 17-year-old Indianapolis high-school student, sought to "take care of things herself" rather than tell her parents that she was pregnant or face a local judge who was known to be anti-abortion. No one knows for sure whether Becky found an illegal abortionist, or if she took some type of drug that caused her to miscarry, but she developed pneumonia and a raging systemic infection, known as *sepsis*, and died in the hospital one week later.[9] Becky's parents, Bill and Karen Bell, and her brother, Bill, Jr., have spearheaded a campaign to repeal parental notification in Indiana, and have traveled to every state that has passed such laws to support similar repeal campaigns.[10]

NEGOTIATING JUDICIAL BYPASS

For many teens, judicial bypass requires missed school days, travel to another town, interaction with numerous strangers and court officials or with adults who know their parents, thus violating their right to confidentiality. An ACLU report documents this judicial travesty. "Public defenders in Duluth [Minn.] represented minors who were the children of their co-workers and in one case had to represent a judge's niece, who waited in the bathroom of the courthouse until her hearing so she would not be recognized.[11] This report also notes that the court proceeding is often so wrenching that some young women have fainted or vomited while waiting for their hearings.[12]

When Tamar, a high school student in Duluth, got pregnant, she told her boyfriend, Stuart, and together they decided that she should have an abortion.

My mother is against abortion, and we decided to go to Minneapolis so she wouldn't find out. We didn't know anything about parental notification, but we found out when we got to the clinic in Minneapolis. The clinic couldn't do an abortion without the notification of both parents because I was 17. I have no relationship with my father, because he raped me when I was 16. I pressed charges and he is now in prison. Since I couldn't get an abortion in Minneapolis, we decided to go back to Duluth and tell Stuart's mother, who might help us to go through the judicial bypass process. Two days later, Stuart, his mother, a counselor from a clinic in Duluth, and I went to the court. I nearly died. The last time I was in that building, it was to convict my father, and it brought the whole nightmare back. When I started to tell my story in court, the public defender who was appointed to represent me turned white and blurted out, "I can't defend you. I'm representing your father on appeal!" That's the first I'd heard about the appeal. The judge requested another lawyer, and my abortion was approved, but I was so upset that I just couldn't go to the clinic. I went to therapy for months, and by the time I got things sorted out, it was too late to have the abortion.

Tamar's case is extreme in its details, but is emblematic of the appalling burdens that parental consent laws impose on young women. Clearly, parental consent laws, which are meant to discourage young women from having abortions, often serve to increase their isolation, impose an even greater economic burden, and increase health risks by causing them to have later abortions; not infrequently, the result is that young women carry their pregnancies to term unwillingly. Parental consent laws also discriminate against young women by holding them responsible for the consequences of sexual activity, without addressing the responsibility of young men in sex and pregnancy, and by requiring young women to answer to their parents or to the courts for their sexual behavior. Unless these laws are repealed, there will be more deaths like those of Becky Bell and Spring Adams, and many more lives will be changed forever, like Tamar's.

Since parental notification laws vary from state to state, it's important to get as much as information as you can about the situation in your state before proceeding. For example, some states have such laws, but they are not enforced, i.e., a sympathetic clinic may accept a note saying that you have permission for an abortion, without checking any further. *Don't do anything crazy! Even though the judicial bypass mechanism is difficult, with proper information and support, many young women have negotiated it successfully.*

Altogether, 39 states have some kind of parental consent/notification laws on the books, only 21 enforce them, and most of these also provide a judicial bypass mechanism.

In 12 states, the laws are being challenged in court and cannot be enforced until the cases are settled. Six states have laws, but do not enforce them.

STATES THAT HAVE PARENTAL CONSENT OR NOTIFICATION LAWS*

The following 21 states require parental consent or notification:

CONSENT

ONE PARENT
Alabama (bypass)
Indiana (bypass)
Louisiana (bypass)
Michigan (bypass)
Missouri (bypass)
Rhode Island (bypass)
South Carolina (parent
or grandparent; bypass)
Wisconsin (parent or
adult family member)
South Carolina
Wisconsin
Wyoming

TWO PARENTS
Massachusetts
(exceptions for 2 parent
requirement; bypass)
North Dakota
(exceptions for 2 parent
requirement; bypass)

NOTIFICATION

ONE PARENT
Arkansas (bypass;
48-hour wait)
Georgia (bypass)
Kansas (bypass)
Nebraska (bypass)
Ohio (bypass;
24-hour wait)
West Virginia (bypass)

TWO PARENTS
Minnesota
(bypass; 48-hour wait)
Utah (2 parent,but one
deemed agent of other;
no bypass)

*This list was developed by the American Civil Liberties Union Reproductive Freedom Project. Used by permission.

The following 12 states have parental consent or notification laws that are being challenged in the courts and cannot be enforced until the cases have been decided:

ONE PARENT
Arizona (bypass)
California (bypass)
Colorado (bypass
or husband)
Florida (bypass)
Pennsylvania (bypass)
Washington (husband
or guardian)

ONE PARENT
Illinois (bypass)
Maryland (doctor may
waive notice if not in
the woman's best
interest)
Nevada (bypass)

TWO PARENTS
Kentucky (bypass)
Mississippi (exceptions
for 2 parent requirement;
bypass)
Tennessee (bypass)

TWO PARENTS

The following six states have laws requiring parental consent/notification of one or both parents that are generally not enforced, and provide no bypass mechanism:

ONE PARENT
Alaska (no bypass)
Delaware (no bypass)
New Mexico (no bypass)
South Dakota (no bypass)

ONE PARENT
Montana (no bypass)

TWO PARENTS

TWO PARENTS
Idaho (no bypass)

Connecticut requires counseling, but not notification, and Maine requires counseling and consent of one adult family member, but provides a bypass mechanism.

INFORMATION FOR WOMEN WHO ARE HIV-POSITIVE OR WHO HAVE AIDS

Although official U.S. government policy established by the Centers for Disease Control encourages women who are HIV-positive or who have been diagnosed with AIDS to postpone pregnancy, these women have the same right to make their own decisions about continuing or terminating a pregnancy as other women do. It is ironic, then, that while many doctors and clinics encourage HIV-positive women to terminate their pregnancies, many clinics across the country have routinely refused to do abortions for women they knew or suspected carried the AIDS virus.

Legally, clinics cannot refuse to do abortions for women who are HIV-positive (as long as the pregnancy is within the clinic's stated range for termination), nor can they employ extraordinary measures such as reporting your HIV status to health officials, subjecting you to judgmental or abusive counseling, or charging you more for the procedure. If you encounter any such discriminatory practices in a clinic or doctor's office, the WHEP *Abortion Guide*[13] recommends reporting it to your city's office of human rights or to an AIDS organization. Reporting such incidents can be useful. In 1990, for example, the New York City Commission on Human Rights publicly investigated clinics that engaged in such practices. As a result of the investigation, clinics that had been singled out agreed to follow established guidelines.

"A woman who is HIV-positive has the right to reveal or not to reveal her HIV status in any situation," says Marion Banzhaf, Director of the New Jersey Women and AIDS Project. Banzhaf points out that, in some instances, a woman who reveals her HIV-positive status may be denied services, or treated in a condescending or disrespectful way by abortion providers. However, acknowledging that you have HIV, ARC, or AIDS reminds doctors and clinic personnel to use standard protective measures. (Known as "universal precautions," these are guidelines to control the transmission of disease, including using protective garments such as gloves, glasses and gowns, handling blood products and spills carefully, disposing of needles in puncture proof containers, and maintaining antiseptic conditions.) These guidelines apply to *all* communicable conditions and may help you get better health care as well. For example, your provider can make sure that the thermometer you use has a sheath, to protect you from infection, and can make efforts to see that you are not directly exposed to communicable diseases by staff or other patients. Knowing that you are HIV-positive could also be crucial in the unlikely event of a complication, especially from a second trimester abortion (see pages 89-93).

Abortion for women who are HIV-positive is no different than for other women, but there a few factors you might want to consider in making your decision whether to have an abortion. Being pregnant normally does not speed the progress of AIDS-related disorders. However, if you decide to carry your pregnancy to term, your baby has a 25 to 30% percent chance of being infected with HIV. If you decide to have an abortion, having general anesthesia might increase your risk of contracting AIDS-related conditions because anesthesia temporarily suppresses the immune system. In abortions after 18 weeks, the risk of anemia is somewhat higher because of greater blood loss during and after the procedure. If you are taking AZT, you may be predisposed toward anemia, which could arise or be worsened by normal blood loss from a second trimester abortion. Therefore, you may want to take preventive steps ahead of time, such as eating plenty of green leafy vegetables, raisins, or beets, or taking iron supplements, vitamins B_6, B_{12}, or folic acid supplements.

PICKETERS AT ABORTION CLINICS

In the past decade, untold numbers of women have had to thread their way through hordes of anti-abortion protesters in order to get their abortions. These picketers cost taxpayers thousands of dollars in law enforcement costs and usually get top billing on prime-time news, but clinic administrators don't believe that they actually prevent many abortions. However, many clinic counselors have noted that they do make women feel guilty about having their abortions, especially young women who may not have a lot of self-confidence.

Women who need abortions have various ways of dealing with picketers. Some choose to ignore them,

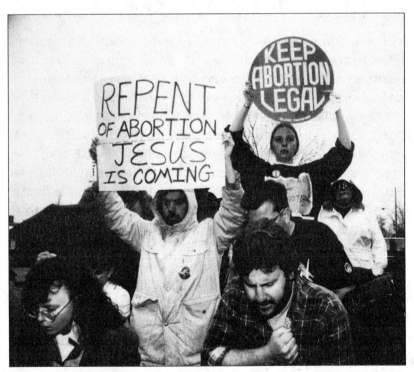

PICKETERS at an abortion clinic in Buffalo, N.Y., in April, 1992.

walking quickly through picket lines with eyes averted, but most react in righteous anger. It is not recommended that you stop and enter into discussion with the picketers.

Picketers often attempt to invade clinics to harass women in waiting rooms or to stop abortions, and they are always taken off by the police in due course. Many are professional picketers who are well aware of the limits of legal behavior—they can't legally touch you or physically block your way into the clinic—but they are always testing these limits if the police are not present or are not looking. Often it is not the police, but volunteer clinic escorts, usually dedicated pro-choice activists, who are the most helpful in preserving women's rights and in keeping "antis" on the street and out of clinic waiting rooms.

PICKETERS GET *THEIR* ABORTIONS

The phenomenon that perhaps best exposes the underlying hypocrisy of the anti-abortion movement is the very common occurrence of women who profess to be staunchly anti-abortion yet show up on the doorsteps of clinics as clients. Variations on this theme include men who accompany their daughters, wives, or girlfriends to the same clinics they regularly picket, and female anti-abortion activists who lay down their picket signs long enough to get their own abortions. These incidents have been common gossip among abortion providers for years, but have been difficult to document because of the reluctance of clinic personnel to breech the confidentiality of their patients, even those who are actively trying to put them out of business.

"Women who think that abortion is wrong, but decide to get one anyway, represent about 15% of our patients," says Sylvia Stengle, founder and director of the Allentown Women's Center in Allentown, Pennsylvania.

"Picketers who get abortions are a small subset of this population."

Sometimes anti-abortion activists attempt to hide their affiliations and activities, but others seem compelled to acknowledge them. **Bernadette, a counselor at an abortion clinic in Texas reports one such incident:**

One day when I was on the front desk, a woman walked in to the clinic to make an appointment. From her behavior, I guessed that she had just come from the anti-abortion 'counseling center' across the street where they try to convince, cajole, or terrorize women into continuing their pregnancies. The woman appeared numb, almost in a state of shock, and in a voice so low that it was almost a whisper, she said that she wanted an abortion. I didn't pressure her for information, but she seemed driven to confess that she had marched with the "pro-life" advocates at City Hall on the recent anniversary of the Roe v. Wade *decision on January 22. She said she was separated from her husband, and that the father was another man, who now had another girlfriend, who was also pregnant. "There's just no way I can have this baby," she told me. Then, gesturing to the other women in the waiting room, she said, "I guess you shouldn't say anything until you are in these women's shoes." Her situation was such a mess. I was torn between sympathy for her, and wagging my finger at her and saying, "Aren't you glad abortion is still legal?"*

Debi Jackson, the administrator of Cincinnati Woman's Services, an abortion clinic in Cincinnati, Ohio, recalls two incidents at her clinic in which fathers who were

**active picketers of the local Planned Parenthood clinic
brought their daughters in for abortions:**

> *Before I came to Cincinnati Woman's Services, I
> was head clinic escort at Planned Parenthood for
> two and one-half years. After all that time, I had
> the faces of the regular picketers memorized.
> Within the first few months on the job, I was
> shocked when one, and then a second male pick-
> eter brought their teenage daughters in for abor-
> tions. Neither apparently realized I had changed
> jobs, but they were both clearly shocked to see
> me. In my experience, these are people who can't
> face having the neighbors or people at church find
> out that their daughters are sexually active. They
> also seem to believe that their daughters are dif-
> ferent from the other women in the waiting room,
> and the daughters seem to think so too. However,
> in the counseling session, we make it clear that
> their behavior, and their predicament, is no dif-
> ferent than that of the clinic's other clients. This
> seems to come as a shock to some of them.*

**Doctors who do abortions also report encountering anti-
abortion activists. Dr. Bruce Steir, who has done abortions in Northern California for many years, describes an
abortion he did for a committed anti-abortion activist:**

> *At a Super Bowl party in San Francisco, I
> observed my daughter-in-law's best friend admon-
> ishing the women who were pro-choice for sup-
> porting "baby killers" (I guess I was one of those
> she had in mind). She stated that she was proud
> to be a "pro-life" activist and Operation Rescue
> supporter. Three months later I entered the oper-
> ating room of a San Francisco abortion clinic and*

*found this same woman sitting on the exam table.
I decided not to remind her of any of her passion-
ately stated convictions. She, however, blew her
cool by timidly confessing that she was still anti-
abortion, saying, "I'm a single working girl and
can't afford maternity clothes, let alone obstetric
care!" There were many words I would like to
have said to her at that moment, but instead I
skillfully did her abortion and left it at that.*

Sylvia Stengle, whose Pennsylvania clinic has been picketed almost weekly since 1978, sees anti-abortion activists
who seek abortions as suffering from something far worse
than a double standard. "Terminating a pregnancy throws
these women into deep emotional conflict. They have to
rationalize their actions, but can't, because they are living
by a dysfunctional value system that doesn't allow for realistic solutions. They are left with guilt and damaged self-
esteem that comes back to haunt them.

"Women who are against abortion often say that
they regret their decision to have one, and many claim
they were pressured into it by husbands, boyfriends, or
parents, or complain that counselors did not provide them
with enough information," Stengle continues. She feels
these "regrets" really represent a failure to take individual
responsibility for the decision to terminate a pregnancy. At
the Allentown clinic, Stengle has developed a special consent form to deal with these women. The form, which has
been adapted by other clinics, requires women who believe
abortion is wrong to acknowledge that they have been
informed of alternatives to abortion, and that they are per-
sonally taking responsibility for ending their pregnancies.
In addition, women who refuse to concede that abortion
should be available to other women must relinquish their
rights to confidentiality. "These women can still get their
abortions, but if we see them back on the picket lines, we

reserve the right to release their names to the media," says Stengle. "This makes them think twice about their decision."

Some clinics do special counseling with women who are vocally against abortion, but reserve the right to refuse to do the procedure in some instances. "After counseling, if a woman still insists that abortion should not be available to other women, and calls us murderers, and so forth, they just have to get their abortions elsewhere," says Lynn Thogersen, Clinic Administrator of the Atlanta Feminist Women's Health Center. The Atlanta clinic has been picketed regularly since 1985, and was severely damaged by anti-abortion protesters in 1989. "Our counselors feel we have to draw the line somewhere."

Female anti-abortion activists who get abortions are the dirty little secret of the anti-abortion movement. Some actually believe they are committing "murder," yet the minute their periods are late, they experience what it means to be unable to control their own reproductive lives. So they grit their teeth, have abortions to avoid having their lives dramatically altered, and often return to the picket lines to try to prevent other women from exercising the same freedom.

COMPARISON SHOPPING

Unfortunately, after deciding to get an abortion, many women call a few places to check the prices, then often choose the cheapest one, even though it may be only $5 or $10 cheaper, without taking any other factors into consideration. As with any service, medical or otherwise, making the right decision about where to get your abortion can be facilitated by getting a direct referral from someone who has used the service you are considering. This is usually the most dependable means of getting good treatment. A positive referral from a friend, relative, doctor, or professional counselor can often help you make a decision and feel confident that it is a good one. If you do not have a direct referral, you can still make the best of what is available by asking specific questions on the phone. Vague or incomplete answers to questions may be indicative of less than adequate care. **Whether checking by phone or in person, you might want to ask:**

➡️ How long will it take to get an appointment?

➡️ How long will I be at the clinic on the day of my abortion?

➡️ How many visits will I have to make?

➡️ Will I have a choice between general and local anesthesia? (See page 79 for more information on the differences between local and general anesthesia.)

➡️ What will the cost be? (See pages 13-15 for information on the costs of an abortion.)

➡️ Is the clinic (or doctor) a member of the National Abortion Federation (NAF)? Because NAF sets standards for abortion care and investigates complaints, membership in NAF is definitely a plus. You can verify a practitioner's membership in NAF by calling 800-772-9100 in the U.S.; 800-424-2280 in Canada; or 202-667-5881 in Washington, D.C.

➡️ What type of procedure is used? (The safest early abortion procedure is *suction* or *aspiration* under local anesthesia, or using no anesthesia at all. Some doctors, and a few clinics, still use *suction curettage*, a combination of the suction procedure and a D&C, but this procedure is considered to be outdated by many abortion experts.)

➡️ To what week of pregnancy does the clinic (or doctor) do abortions? (This is a very important question, especially if you are more than 12 weeks pregnant and/or you must travel to another town or state for your abortion. Many clinics, including Planned Parenthood, only do abortions up to 12, or at the outside, 16 weeks from the last normal menstrual period.)

➡ Will a counselor be present during the procedure?

➡ Can I bring a friend with me, and can he or she be in the procedure room with me?

➡ Where will I be sent if emergency follow-up is needed?

SEXUAL HARASSMENT

In illegal situations, and on occasion in legal ones, there have been reports of women who have been taken advantage of sexually as a sort of "additional charge" for an abortion. **If you find yourself in a situation where you sense an atmosphere of sexual harassment, there are some self-defense strategies that may help**:

➡ Be alert for any suggestive remarks by the practitioner.

➡ Undress only as needed. Your vagina and uterus are the only parts of your body that need to be examined for an abortion, i.e., you don't need to take your blouse and bra off. (You may be required to disrobe and wear a gown if you are having general anesthesia.)

➡ Report any incident of sexual harassment to your state medical board or to the National Abortion Federation (800-772-9100).

FINDING A SYMPATHETIC DOCTOR
TO DO AN ABORTION

In the days before abortion was legal, women could often get abortions if they had an acceptable medical reason, such as an impending miscarriage, "menstrual irregularities," a pregnancy that was the result of rape or incest, serious problems with alcohol or drug abuse, symptoms of mental illness, or if they threatened to attempt suicide or self-abortion. Doctors who were opposed to abortion typically refused to perform procedures on the basis of such problems, but sympathetic doctors readily used any excuse, no matter how flimsy, to do what came in late pre-*Roe* days to be called "therapeutic abortions."

Surveys have shown that the vast majority of doctors, especially women doctors, are pro-choice. Therefore, if you consult a doctor about an unintended pregnancy, even if he or she does not do abortions, there is a substantial likelihood that you will get help in some way. The exception to this may be Catholic doctors, or doctors who are affiliated with Catholic hospitals.

Today, even in states where there are severe restrictions on abortion, often there are certain circumstances in which abortions can still be done, such as rape, incest, or particular medical or psychiatric conditions that might endanger the fetus or the life of a pregnant woman. In some cases, a fetus may be aborted if a woman has been directly exposed to environmental hazards such as lead, mercury, or high-dose X-rays, if she has taken certain prescription medications, or even street drugs such as crack cocaine, known to cause fetal abnormalities (teratogenic effects) in early pregnancy, or if she has a current problem with alcohol or drug abuse.

In areas where abortion is illegal or unavailable, many women travel to another town or state, but this takes time, and depending on the distance, can be expensive. Women who find travel unacceptable often seek out sympathetic doctors in their own communities who might do abortions for them quietly, without fanfare, or on some excuse that is acceptable under the particular laws or regulations of the state. Given a strong enough reason, i.e., a believable threat to commit suicide or to self-abort, even an unsympathetic doctor may be convinced to do an abortion.

Yet, because of the anti-abortion climate at the hospital where they have admitting privileges, or in the community in general, some doctors who are sympathetic may be afraid to terminate a pregnancy without a very compelling reason. They may fear—and reasonably so—that they will be in danger of losing hospital privileges or being arrested if it is discovered that they did an abortion.

A DOCTOR'S ETHICAL AND LEGAL RESPONSIBILITY

Every doctor, regardless of his or her personal beliefs, is required by ethical standards to treat any medical emergency. If you are refused treatment for a threatened miscarriage or for an incomplete abortion, regardless of how it was started, or if signs of mental illness, especially of threatened suicide, are not taken seriously, you—or your family if you die—may have grounds for a malpractice lawsuit against the doctor and/or hospital.

The next several sections describe various ruses that women have used—and will no doubt use again—to get abortions, in areas where abortion is inaccessible or illegal.

FAKING A MISCARRIAGE

Miscarriages are common, occurring in an estimated 15% of all pregnancies (about one in six), but early miscarriages are often mistaken for a menstrual period and go unreported, so this figure could be considerably higher. In fact, some endocrinologists believe that 50% of fertilized eggs are never implanted and are eliminated. After about eight to 10 weeks, however, the symptoms of an impending miscarriage are quite distinct: cramps that come in waves which can be period-like or fairly intense, heavy bleeding, which may or may not be accompanied by pain, large clots or bits of wispy tissue, weakness, faintness, dizziness, and nausea.

In the past, women often got abortions by faking a miscarriage, claiming waves of cramps, fainting episodes (the more dramatic the better), and exhibiting blood on their underwear or clothes. Today, however, due to advances in sonography, an imaging system that employs high frequency sound waves to produce a visible X-ray-like picture (see page 75), the fetal heartbeat can now be detected as early as five to six weeks from the last menstrual period, so if a doctor or clinic has access to sonography equipment, getting an abortion because of a threatened miscarriage isn't as easy as it used to be. In addition, blood pregnancy tests can now detect the amount of pregnancy hormone in the urine, and provide rather precise information about the progress or decline of a pregnancy as early as seven to 10 days after conception.

Nonetheless, a sympathetic doctor may be won over by convincing signs of a miscarriage, and may be willing to "finish it," especially in rural or isolated areas, which more closely duplicate conditions in pre-*Roe* days, when medical care was much less standardized. With skillfully written notes on a woman's chart, it would be difficult for anyone to tell, after the fact, that completing a miscarriage wasn't necessary.

Jenny, a retired reporter from a small town in Idaho, successfully faked a miscarriage in the late 1960s.

I was 35, not married, and liked my work. Children just weren't in the picture, nor was my boyfriend, for that matter. I didn't know what to do, but told Juliette, my best friend, who was a nurse, and she told me about her own miscarriage. Being a reporter, I asked her a lot of questions, and we figured out how I could fake a miscarriage and get a D&C. Juliette drew some of my blood just before I went to the hospital on

Friday night about 10:00. She also gave me a bottle of her urine, which would test negative on the "rabbit test," as they called pregnancy tests back then. A negative urine test might indicate that a miscarriage was occurring. When I got to the emergency room, before I went to the registration desk, I went into the bathroom and poured one tube of blood on a sanitary pad, which I had worn, being careful to get a good bit on my slip and skirt as well. When I undressed, I made sure that my clothes were arranged with the blood clearly visible. When I saw the doctor, I told him that my period was about five weeks late, that I had been spotting lightly for about two weeks. I told him that when I woke up that morning, I had begun bleeding rather heavily and had to change my pad every two or three hours, and that I had seen some clots in the toilet, which looked more stringy than the ones I occasionally had with my period. I told him I had started to feel faint while I was cooking supper, and felt so nauseous I couldn't eat, and decided to come to the hospital. He took this all very seriously and asked me if I was having any cramping. "It comes and goes, and about every half hour, it gets stronger," I said. Then he put a thermometer in my mouth and, of course, left for 20 minutes. While he was out, making sure no one was looking, I walked over to the sink and ran some warm water on the thermometer until the temperature reached 100°. When the doctor came back in, he took one look at the thermometer and said, "Well, young lady, I think you need a D&C."

Jenny was never sure whether the doctor believed her story, but thinks that her own blood and an elevated temperature were probably the keys to a successful act.

Of course, there are many variables to faking a miscarriage, and many places where a carefully devised plan can fall apart. Today, with a positive pregnancy test and the absence of an elevated temperature, many doctors would probably send a woman home for a couple of days to wait and see what happens. Women need to be creative and must be prepared to improvise on the spot depending on the variables of the situation.

FAKING RAPE

Before abortion was legal, women sometimes got abortions by claiming that they had been raped, but like faking a miscarriage, this scheme was fraught with vagaries and uncertainties.

Belinda, an artist who lived in Miami in the late 1950s, tells her story:

> *Three successive doctors refused to help me, and I was getting pretty discouraged. Finally, the fourth one, a woman, said, "If you had been raped, I could do a D&C." That's all she said, but I got the message, and thought about what to do. The next morning, I went to my local precinct and said that a month ago, a man forced me into his car at knifepoint in the parking lot of the grocery store just as it closed and that he drove to a secluded area by a canal and forced me to have sex in the back seat. I told the sergeant that I was too scared to fight, and that when he was driving around afterward I noticed that the door handle was*

missing—most likely removed. The sergeant liked that little detail a lot, and started to get interested. He was very annoyed that I had waited a whole month to report such a serious incident, but I said it had taken me that long to get up the nerve to do it, and he seemed to accept that. In spite of the time lapse, he wanted me to have a medical examination, so I asked if I could be seen by my own doctor, and he agreed. So I went back to the doctor I had seen earlier with a copy of the police report. After having a positive pregnancy test, she sent me to a psychiatrist, and both of them submitted reports to a hospital committee and recommended that I get an abortion.

Only in desperate situations—such as women may find themselves in in the future if states ban abortions except for certain reasons such as rape—should women even consider resorting to faking rape. Doing so has the potential to undermine the gains of the movement against violence against women which has worked to overcome the myth used by hostile prosecutors and judges that women who report rape cannot be trusted. However, a time and place can be envisioned where a woman, her doctor, and sympathetic authorities would be forced to go through a charade of a rape complaint about some unknown, unidentifiable assailant in order to get around hypocritical, restrictive laws. This charade would be clearly recognized by all participants and it would bear little resemblance to the real thing, a genuine rape complaint.

At present, outright bans on abortion have been passed by two state legislatures, Utah and Louisiana, and the possession of Guam, but these laws have been challenged and cannot be enforced until they are upheld by the Supreme Court. Most constitutional law experts do not expect these laws to be upheld.

FAKING MENTAL ILLNESS

In pre-*Roe* days in many states, "mental illness" became one of the medically acceptable reasons that allowed a woman to get a D&C at her local hospital. Usually one or more psychiatrists had to certify that she had some "borderline" mental condition that might become worse if the pregnancy continued or, in extreme cases, that a woman might become a "danger" to herself or to others. These were highly subjective judgment calls and psychiatrists usually had great leeway in how they assessed a woman's condition.[14]

In *The Abortion Handbook*,[15] Lana Phelan and Pat Maginnis encourage women to take full advantage of mental health provisions in abortion laws. **The *Handbook*'s tongue-in-cheek scenario is somewhat overstated, but provides an idea of how a woman might go about convincing a therapist that she has more pressing things to deal with than having a baby:**

> *During the interview...weep, show anger, fear, disgust, outright destructiveness of your clothing or small objects, say, the ashtray on his desk which can be broken on the floor or against a wall. Don't overdo this. You will be billed for the broken things later! Don't break the doctor's head. This is a "no-no"...How's your attention span?...You can't seem to concentrate on anything for more than a couple of minutes...Drop sly hints that you are "attracted" to many strange men sexually. Be dull and very sad. Cry a bit. Just sit in silence, and make him repeat questions as though you hadn't heard a word...And now for the Manic Scene: Just like opera, ladies! Brighten up, beam like a sunrise...let your thoughts gallop wildly...your*

speech flows like the Danube in flood time...You might try taking off your shoes, kicking them all the way across his office, wriggling your toes. Then say, "That feels so good, I think I'll take everything off...(musingly)."

What the authors are suggesting here is faking manic depression, now referred to as a "bi-polar" disorder. Realistically, people with bi-polar disorders don't exhibit both mania and depression in the same 50-minute session. Some people experience only, or primarily, manic behavior, which gets worse at times. Others may be chronically depressed most of the time. Some people exhibit both poles (hence the term bi-polar) at different times, in phases that last several weeks to several months. Classic signs of depression that any therapist ought to pick up on are a decline in interest in personal appearance, fatigue, changes in appetite, weight loss, sleep disturbances, mood swings, fatigue, lack of ability to concentrate, outbursts of temper, decreased functioning in everyday activities (e.g., missing work, school, or important appointments), increased alcohol or drug use, and morbid thought patterns. In the manic phase, people often feel exuberant, thoughts may race, and speech might be accelerated. Some people take on overly ambitious projects, spend money wildly, and experience increased sexual desire. In both the manic and the depressive phases, many people have several prominent symptoms, and perhaps several that are less pronounced—but not all possible symptoms at once.[16]

Having a history of depression, suicidal thoughts, or drug abuse can also be helpful in convincing a therapist of the need for an abortion. Sometimes former therapists are willing to embellish records a bit to add weight to a request for an abortion on psychiatric grounds. If a therapist thinks your life may go down the drain at the nearest liquor store or crack house, he or she might be willing to write a strong letter on your behalf to a hospital committee or whoever approves "medically necessary" abortions.

THREATENING SUICIDE

Another pre-*Roe* standby that many women employed successfully was threatening or feigning suicide. Sadly, some women weren't just feigning. (See Dr. Ruth Barnett's poignant account of one of her young patients on pages 101-102.) Because of the grave nature of such threats, medical ethics require that doctors and therapists take them seriously.

Annie, a college student in Gainesville, Florida, in 1963, who is now a doctor in Nebraska, told us how she succeeded in convincing a rather reluctant psychiatrist to help her get an abortion:

> *I had been secretly sleeping with my boyfriend off campus for several months, and just after spring vacation, began to suspect that I was pregnant. I knew other girls were having sex, but few talked about it openly. I had no idea of what to do. I had my heart set on going to medical school, but I knew that women who went to medical school didn't have babies. As the weeks passed, I got depressed and started skipping classes. One day I had such a headache that I took four aspirin, the last ones in the bottle, and fell asleep. When my roommate came in, she tried to wake me up to tell me about the test I had just missed, but I was so depressed, I just groaned and turned back over. Then she found the empty aspirin bottle, and in a panic called the dorm supervisor, who overreacted and called the ambulance, police, and the school*

psychiatrist. I was feeling really angry, and out of spite, told them that I didn't know how many aspirin were in the bottle, but that I had taken them all. I was taken to the hospital, where my stomach was pumped, but they didn't get anything. The resident who put the tube in my nose remarked that it was a good thing I hadn't taken any "real pills." Afterward I began to think: if they can do all of this over a few aspirin, what will they do if I take "real pills"? I had no idea what "real pills" were, but I knew a girl in my roommate's sorority named Nancy who always took a lot of pills. Her cousin was a pharmacist in Jacksonville who got them for her, and she had a special little suitcase that she kept them in. I told Nancy that I needed a bottle and a couple of pills to play a trick on the school psychiatrist, whom I was now required to visit. I saw him as my only hope for getting an abortion, and I didn't want to blow it. She gave me a bottle and a couple of red oval tablets. "These will shake him up a bit," Nancy said knowingly. From there, I went to the drugstore and found some iron pills that were roughly the same size and color as the pills Nancy gave me. Before my appointment I drank some rum and thought about my plan. Since I really didn't know what I was up against, I decided to play it cool. During my appointment, I told the psychiatrist that I was sure I was pregnant and wanted an abortion, and he started giving me a lecture about how I was ruining my life, and so forth, and that you had to a have reason to get an abortion. I started to cry, and casually reached into my purse and put the pill bottle on the table between us. He took the bait and picked up the bottle and asked me where I had gotten the pills. "From a friend," I

> *answered innocently. "What are you going to do with them?" he asked, a little alarmed. "I'm going to buy a bottle of rum and take all of them," I said, surprised at my own boldness. He took the pills and put them in his pocket and tried to get me to tell him who had given them to me. We started arguing and I got mad and told him I could get more—a lot more—at any time. At that point, he was hooked. He got on the phone to the hospital and arranged to admit me, then asked his secretary to drive me to the hospital. I was registered as a regular patient, but put in the psychiatric ward, and the next morning I had a D&C.*

When unsympathetic doctors have refused to help, some women have found that threatening suicide, or by threatening to do their abortion themselves has gotten quick action in getting a therapeutic abortion arranged. Without proper information, self-abortion is very risky and often doesn't work. However, many doctors and therapists will do whatever needs to be done to arrange a legal abortion, either locally, or in another location, when threatened with the alternative of a self-abortion.

DIAGNOSTIC TESTS
SIMILAR TO AN ABORTION

Terminating a pregnancy is not the only reason the contents of the uterus are removed. There are diagnostic tests for menstrual irregularities, uterine cancer, and other uterine abnormalities, called *endometrial biopsies*, in which the lining of the uterus, the *endometrium*, and any menstrual blood are removed by suction and examined in a laboratory. These two- to three-minute office procedures can be done with a hand-operated syringe such as the International Projects Assistance Services (IPAS)[17] kit (see illustration on page 124), or with a mechanical aspirator used for an abortions. Some gynecologists still use the D&C technique for these simple procedures because it is what they are used to, although it requires general anesthesia and is slightly more risky than the vacuum techniques.

One of the primary reasons endometrial biopsies are done is for so-called "dysfunctional bleeding," a condition associated primarily with menopause, that can occur in younger women as well. The ambiguous term is often used by doctors to describe exceptionally heavy or unpredictable menstrual periods. Generally, such bleeding is just a normal readjustment to changing levels of hormones, but sometimes it can signal uterine cancer. Doctors usually monitor such bleeding for several months, however if they suspect cancer for any reason, especially if you complain of episodic, heavy bleeding that started suddenly and has continued for several months, an endometrial biopsy may be recommended.

Most doctors will do a pregnancy test before doing a biopsy, but if an abnormality is suspected, the biopsy may have to be done anyway. In any event, uterine aspirations for diagnostic purposes are done solely at the discretion of a doctor, are easy to justify, and are not likely to be questioned.

"If abortion becomes illegal in Massachusetts, I plan to do a lot more endometrial biopsies," one prominent Boston gynecologist told us, meaning that he will do abortions under the guise of diagnostic procedures. He also noted that many of his colleagues had expressed similar intentions.

HAZARDS OF THE EMERGENCY ROOM

Women who have gone to the emergency room with a miscarriage in progress, especially if it was deliberately induced, have found that they need to be very careful what they say there. Some doctors, nurses, or other health care professionals are anti-abortion and are prone to give moralistic lectures, treat women disrespectfully, and even threaten to turn them over to the police. *The Abortion Handbook* **has some sage advice for women who must endure such insults:**

> *Grit your teeth. Give your name and address only, and yell for a lawyer. If they threaten to withhold medical care, threaten to sue or have your heirs sue if they let you die...Before seeing the doctor...look behind all doors and furniture for nurse types, and then ask the physician to keep your medical confidence as he has sworn to do. Tell him if he reports you to the police, you will not talk to them until you have a lawyer present. Then tell the doctor the absolute truth...If someone has helped you, tell him what method they used, but you do not have to tell him their names.*[18]

Although many Catholic doctors and nurses are pro-choice, or at least are not rabidly anti-abortion, many women have reported being rudely treated at Catholic hospitals, as well as at non-Catholic hospitals by nurses or other hospital staff who are anti-abortion, when they seek treatment for an abortion complication. Therefore, if you have a miscarriage or abortion complication, it might be wise to avoid going to Catholic hospitals if you have a choice.

DON'T TAKE "NO" FOR AN ANSWER

Making use of the NAF Hotline, the information networks listed in Chapter 2, loopholes in abortion laws, and doctors' considerable leeway in what they do in private practice, almost every woman will be able to get an abortion if she needs or wants one.

CHAPTER TWO

Information Networks

IN RESPONSE to increasing restrictions on abortion, a nationwide network of groups is evolving to help women obtain safe abortions and to do the legal and legislative work necessary to keep abortion legal. **These groups include:**

➡ WOMEN'S HEALTH PROJECTS (page 53), a loose-knit network of feminist abortion clinics such as the Federation of Feminist Women's Health Centers, the Vermont and New Hampshire Feminist Health Centers, the Emma Goldman Clinic for Women, and the Elizabeth Blackwell Clinic for Women, and numerous smaller women's health projects. In addition, a host of women's health projects such as the Boston Women's Health Book Collective (the authors of *Our Bodies, Ourselves*), the Women's Health Education Project in New York City, and the Bay Area Coalition for Reproductive Rights (BACORR) are dedicated to providing information on women's health concerns, but with a special emphasis on reproductive health issues.

➡ NATIONAL FEMINIST, LEGAL, AND PUBLIC POLICY ORGANIZATIONS that support reproductive rights (page 60). These groups, such as the National Abortion Rights Action League (NARAL), the Fund for the Feminist Majority, and the National Women's Health Network, are working on many levels to keep abortion legal. Public policy organizations such as the Alan Guttmacher Institute do research and analysis on abortion, and provide accurate information to the public and the media. Activist legal organizations such as the Center for Reproductive Law and Policy (formerly the Reproductive Freedom Project of the ACLU) do legal research and argue abortion rights cases in the courts.

THE OVERGROUND RAILROAD

The day after the *Webster* decision, July 4, 1989, women at the annual Quaker gathering in Pennsylvania were galvanized into action. "We were so frustrated and angry," says Mary Ellen MacNish, a nurse who works at a Planned Parenthood clinic in Baltimore. "We realized that we were tired of winning the battles, and then having the men in power change the rules." Based on the Quakers' historical participation in the underground railroad that transported slaves to freedom during the struggle for the abolition of slavery, plans emerged for a "Overground Railroad," a network to help transport women to states where abortion is legal, and to provide "safe houses" for them. Already the group has chapters in 23 states.

➡ FINANCIAL ASSISTANCE AND LOAN SOURCES, (see page 62) which provide direct funding to pay for abortions for young, poor, or undocumented women, or make low- or no-interest loans for abortion care. These groups may also provide information on transportation and lodging. Many of these organizations can help you determine if you are eligible for Medicaid in states where those funds are still available, and knowledgeable staff may be able to help you qualify if you are eligible.

➡️ THE NATIONAL ORGANIZATION FOR WOMEN (NOW), which has more than 600 local chapters; each chapter has an abortion task force that is up-to-date on where to obtain abortions. Check the phone directory or call the national NOW office at (202) 331-0066 for the location of the NOW chapter closest to you.

➡️ WOMEN'S CENTERS ON COLLEGE CAMPUSES. Nearly every college campus has a women's center, many of which have task forces on abortion and other reproductive rights issues. They may be able to provide reliable abortion referrals in their communities.

➡️ LOCAL PRO-CHOICE COALITIONS, which may include abortion rights activists, administrators and staff of abortion clinics, professional women, students, housewives, therapists, and social workers. These groups are too

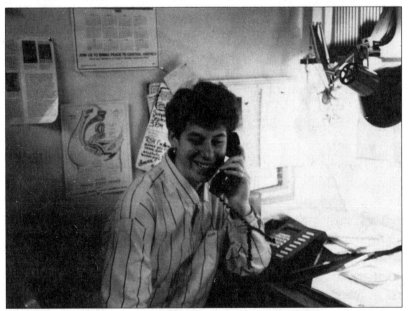

A COUNSELOR at the Elizabeth Black Clinic for Women in Philadelphia responds to questions about the clinic's abortion services.

numerous to be listed here, and may or may not be listed in the phone book, but any one of the groups on these lists is likely to help you identify the pro-choice coalition in your community. If you can find such a group, its members will surely have information on the nearest legal abortion clinic, as well as the names of doctors who are willing to perform abortions.

➡ INTERNATIONAL WOMEN'S HEALTH PROJECT AND INFORMATION CLEARINGHOUSES (page 64). In countries where abortion is illegal or highly restricted, women find abortionists through both official and unofficial sources. In urban areas of foreign countries, sources of information about abortion may include government health services, private voluntary organizations, private non-profit family planning organizations such as the International Planned Parenthood Federation (IPPF), or independent profit-making clinics and doctor's offices. Sometimes these are the same places that actually perform abortions. A variety of women's groups may also operate quite visibly in the cities, and serve as clearinghouses for information on many aspects of women's health, including abortion and childbirth. In rural areas, unofficial sources of abortion information include midwives, nurses and traditional healers. Some clinics operate in rural areas, but there are far too few of these to serve the millions of women who need abortions every year. Even in countries with the most restrictive laws, informal networks of women's groups may have information about local doctors, midwives and other trustworthy practitioners who are willing to do abortions. They may make a direct referral, or take a name and pass it along to a group or practitioner who will then make the contact. To find these groups, you might try contacting the most visible woman-identified organization listed in the telephone book, or contact a national women's department or commission, if one exists. For official reasons, these offices may not make referrals, but often someone in the office who is in contact with groups who will make an abortion referral.

If you call any of the groups on the following lists, you are likely to get a friendly voice on the other end of the phone line, and information on how to find an abortion provider.

WOMEN'S HEALTH PROJECTS

The groups on this list form a loose-knit network of abortion clinics owned and operated by women, community clinics run by and/or for women, and health information and abortion referral projects. Groups that provide abortions are noted by a 🌢. These groups may be very helpful in identifying doctors or clinics that provide abortions in their own communities, and/or provide general information on women's health issues.

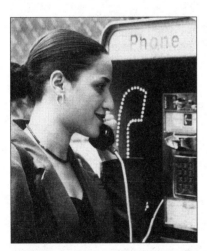

IT MAY TAKE several phone calls before you get the information you need, but keep trying! Someone will help you. [Credit: Nina Berman/SIPA]

CALIFORNIA

BAY AREA HEALING TAO
P.O. Box 460195
San Francisco, CA 94146
(415) 824-3322

BAY AREA COALITION OF
REPRODUCTIVE RIGHTS
(BACORR)
5337 College Ave. #213
Oakland, CA 94618
(510) 541-5690

BERKELEY WOMEN'S HEALTH
CENTER
2908 Ellsworth
Berkeley, CA 94704
(510) 843-6194

BUENA VISTA WOMEN'S
SERVICES
2000 Van Ness St. #406
San Francisco CA 94109
(415) 771-5000

CHICO FEMINIST WOMEN'S
HEALTH CENTER ❧
330 Flume St.
Chico, CA 95926
(916) 891-1911

COALITION FOR THE MEDICAL
RIGHTS OF WOMEN
1638-B Haight St.
San Francisco, CA 94117
(415) 621-8030

COMMITTEE TO DEFEND
REPRODUCTIVE RIGHTS
25 Taylor St. #704
San Francisco CA 94102
(415) 441-4434

DES ACTION
1638-B, Haight St.
San Francisco, CA 94117
(415) 621-8030

GENTLE BIRTH CENTER
116 South Louise St.
Glendale, CA 91205
(818) 545-7128

HAIGHT ASHBURY
FREE CLINIC
Women's Needs Center
1825 Haight St.
San Francisco CA 94117
(415) 221-7371

LESBIAN HEALTH PROJECT
8235 Santa Monica Blvd.
Suite 308
West Hollywood, CA 90046
(213) 650-1508

LYON MARTIN WOMEN'S
HEALTH SERVICES
1748 Market St., Suite 201
San Francisco, CA 94102
(415) 565-7667

NATIONAL LATINA HEALTH
ORGANIZATION
P.O. Box 7567
Oakland CA 94601
(510) 534-1362

NORTHCOUNTRY
CLINIC FOR WOMEN
AND CHILDREN
785 19th St.
Arcata, CA 95521
(707) 822-1385

REDDING FEMINIST WOMEN'S
HEALTH CENTER ❧
1901 Victor Ave.
Redding, CA 96002
(916) 221-0193

SACRAMENTO FEMINIST
WOMEN'S HEALTH CENTER ❧
3701 J St., #201
Sacramento, CA 95816
(916) 451-0621

SANTA CRUZ WOMEN'S
HEALTH CENTER
250 Locust St.
Santa Cruz, CA 95060
(408) 427-3500

SANTA ROSA FEMINIST
WOMEN'S HEALTH CENTER ❧
1144 Montgomery Dr.
Santa Rosa, CA 95405
(707) 575-8212

SPERM BANK OF
CALIFORNIA REPRODUCTIVE
TECHNOLOGIES
Telegraph Hill Medical Plaza
3007 Telegraph Ave., Suite 2
Oakland, CA 94609
(510) 444-2014

WESTSIDE WOMEN'S CLINIC ⊷
1711 Ocean Park Blvd.
Santa Monica, CA 90405
(213) 450-2191

WOMEN'S COMMUNITY CLINIC
696 E. Santa Clara St. #204
San Jose, CA 95112
(408) 287-4090

WHOLISTIC HEALTH
FOR WOMEN
8235 Santa Monica Blvd.
Suite 308
West Hollywood, CA 90046
(213) 650-1508

WOMANCARE, A FEMINIST
WOMEN'S HEALTH CENTER ⊷
2850 6th Ave., Suite 311
San Diego, CA 92103
(619) 298-9352

WEST COAST FEMINIST
HEALTH PROJECT WOMEN'S
CHOICE CLINIC ⊷
2930 McClure St.
Oakland, CA 94609
(510) 444-5676

COLORADO

BOULDER VALLEY WOMEN'S
HEALTH CENTER
2855 Valmont
Boulder, CO 80301
(303) 442-5160

CONNECTICUT

HISPANIC HEALTH COUNCIL
98 Cedar St., #3A
Hartford, CT 06106
(203) 527-0856

WOMEN'S HEALTH
SERVICES ⊷
911 State St.
New Haven, CT 06511
(203) 777-4781

FLORIDA

FEMINIST WOMEN'S HEALTH
CENTER ⊷
505 W. Georgia St.
Tallahassee, FL 32301
(904) 224-9600

GAINESVILLE WOMEN'S
HEALTH CENTER ⊷
720 N.W. 23rd Ave.
Gainesville, FL 32609
(904) 377-5055

GEORGIA

FEMINIST WOMEN'S
HEALTH CENTER
(abortions to 26 weeks)
580 14th St., N.W.
Atlanta, GA 30318
(404) 874-7551

ILLINOIS

CHICAGO WOMEN'S
HEALTH CENTER
3435 N. Sheffield
Chicago, IL 60657
(312) 935-6126

WOMEN ORGANIZED FOR
REPRODUCTIVE CHOICE/
CHICAGO WOMEN'S AIDS
PROJECT
5249 N. Kenmore Ave.
Chicago, IL 60640
(312) 271-2070

WOMEN OF ALL RED
NATIONS (WARN)
4511 N. Hermitage
Chicago, IL 60640

IOWA

CEDAR RAPIDS CLINIC
FOR WOMEN ✿
86 1/2 16th Ave., S.W.
Cedar Rapids, IA 52404
(319) 365-9527

EMMA GOLDMAN CLINIC
FOR WOMEN ✿
715 N. Dodge
Iowa City, IA 52240
(319) 337-2111

MAINE

MABEL WADSWORTH
WOMEN'S HEALTH CENTER
P.O. Box 20
Bangor, ME 04401

MASSACHUSETTS

BOSTON REPRODUCTIVE
RIGHTS NETWORK (R2N2)
P.O. Box 686
Jamaica Plain, MA 02130

BOSTON WOMEN'S HEALTH
BOOK COLLECTIVE
240A Elm St.
Somerville MA 02144
(617) 625-0271

EVERYWOMAN'S CENTER
HEALTH PROJECT
University of Massachusetts
Wilder Hall
Amherst, MA 01003
(413) 545-0883

FENWAY COMMUNITY
HEALTH CENTER
7 Haviland St.
Boston, MA 02115
(617) 267-0900

NEW BEDFORD WOMEN'S
CENTER
252 County St.
New Bedford, MA 02740
(508) 996-3343

REPRODUCTIVE RIGHTS
NETWORK (R2 N2)
P.O. Box 686
Jamaica Plain, MA 02130

WOMEN OF COLOR FOR
REPRODUCTIVE FREEDOM
P.O. Box 1200
Boston, MA 02117-1200

MINNESOTA

PRO-CHOICE RESOURCES
3255 Hennepin Ave. S., #255
Minneapolis, MN 55408
(612) 825-9122

WOMEN'S HEALTH CARE
ASSOCIATION
1455 Lake St., W., #307
Minneapolis, MN 55408
(612) 827-5501

MINNESOTA INDIAN WOMEN'S
RESOURCE CENTER
1900 Chicago Ave.
Minneapolis, MN 55404
(612) 728-2000

MISSOURI

WOMEN'S SELF-HELP CENTER
2838 Olive St.
St. Louis, MO 63103
(314) 531-2003

MONTANA

BLUE MOUNTAIN
WOMEN'S CLINIC ✒
715 Kensington, #24A
Missoula, MT 59801
(406) 721-1646

WOMAN'S PLACE
521 N. Orange
Missoula, MT 59802
(406) 543-7606

NEW HAMPSHIRE

CONCORD FEMINIST
HEALTH CENTER ✒
38 S. Main St.
Concord, NH 03301
(603) 225-2739

THE FEMINIST HEALTH
CENTER OF
PORTSMOUTH ✒
559 Portsmouth Ave.
P.O. Box 456
Greenland, NH 03840
(603) 436-7588

NEW JERSEY

NEW JERSEY RIGHT
TO CHOOSE
Fran Avollone
P.O. Box 343
East Brunswick, NJ 08816
(908) 254-8665

NEW JERSEY WOMEN AND
AIDS NETWORK
5 Elm Row, #112
New Brusnwick NJ 08901
(908) 846-4462

NEW MEXICO

SANTA FE HEALTH
EDUCATION PROJECT
P.O. Box 577
Santa Fe, NM 87504-0557
(505) 982-3236

WOMEN'S HEALTH
SERVICES ✒
505 Early St.
Santa Fe, NM 87501
(505) 988-8869

NEW YORK

FERTILITY AWARENESS
CENTER
P.O. Box 2606
New York, NY 10003
(212) 475-4490

CENTER FOR MEDICAL
CONSUMERS
237 Thompson St.
New York, NY 10012
(212) 674-7105

COMMUNITY HEALTH
PROJECT
Women's Clinic
208 W. 13th St.
New York, NY 10014
(212) 675-3559

HEALTH HOUSE
555 N. Country Rd.
St. James, NY 11780
(516) 862-6743

LOWER EAST SIDE WOMEN'S
CENTER
53 Stanton St.
New York, NY 10002
(212) 353-1924

MATERNITY CENTER
ASSOCIATION
48 E. 92nd St.
New York, NY 10128
(212) 369-7300

REDSTOCKINGS
P.O. Box 744
Stuyvesant Station
New York, NY 10009
(212) 777-9241

ST. MARKS WOMEN'S HEALTH
COLLECTIVE
9 Second Ave.
New York, NY 10003
(212) 228-7482

STUDENTS ORGANIZING
STUDENTS
1600 Broadway, #404
New York NY 10019
(212) 977-6710

WOMANCAP
25 5th Ave., #1A
New York, NY 10003
(212) 529-8489

WOMEN AND AIDS RESOURCE
NETWORK
P.O. Box 20525
Brooklyn, NY 11202

THE WOMEN'S ALTERNATIVE
CLINIC at the State University
of New York at Purchase
735 Anderson Hill Rd.
Purchase, NY 10583
(914) 251-6386

WHAM! (WOMEN'S HEALTH
ACTION AND MOBILIZATION)
P.O. Box 733
New York NY 10009
(212) 713-5966

WOMEN'S HEALTH CENTER
60 Central Ave.
Cortland, NY 13045
(607) 753-5027

WOMEN'S HEALTH
EDUCATION NETWORK
P.O. Box 58
Brooklyn, NY 11222

WOMEN'S HEALTH
EDUCATION PROJECT
P.O. Box 20284
Tompkins Square Station
New York, NY 10009
(212) 633-0946

WOMEN'S LIBERATION FRONT
P.O. Box 1287
Port Ewen, NY 12466

OREGON

PORTLAND WOMEN'S
HEALTH CENTER ⬥
1020 N.E. 2nd Ave.
Suite 200
Portland, OR 97232
(503) 233-0808

PENNSYLVANIA

ELIZABETH BLACKWELL
HEALTH CENTER FOR
WOMEN ⬥
1124 Walnut St.
Philadelphia, PA 19107
(215) 923-7577

RHODE ISLAND

RHODE ISLAND WOMEN'S
HEALTH COLLECTIVE
90 Printery St.
Providence, RI 02906
(401) 861-0030

SOUTH DAKOTA

NATIVE AMERICAN
WOMEN'S HEALTH
Education Resource Center
P.O. Box 572
Lake Andes, SD 57356
(605) 487-7072

VERMONT

SOUTHERN VERMONT
WOMEN'S HEALTH
CENTER ✎
187 N. Main St.
Rutland, VT 05701
(802) 775-1946

VERMONT WOMEN'S HEALTH
CENTER ✎
336 North Ave.
Burlington, VT 05401
(802) 863-1386

WASHINGTON

ARADIA WOMEN'S HEALTH
CENTER ✎
112 Boylston Ave. E.
Seattle WA 98115
(206) 323-9388

CEDAR RIVER CLINIC,
A Feminist Women's
Health Center
4300 Talbot Rd. S., #403
Renton, WA 98055
(206) 255-0471

45TH STREET COMMUNITY
HEALTH CLINIC
1629 N. 45th St.
Seattle, WA 98103
(206) 633-3350

YAKIMA FEMINIST WOMEN'S
HEALTH CENTER ✎
106 E. E St.
Yakima, WA 98901
(509) 575-6422

WASHINGTON, D.C.

WASHINGTON FREE CLINIC
Women's Health Collective
1156 Wisconsin Ave., N.W.
Washington, DC 20007
(202) 667-1106

WEST VIRGINIA

WOMEN'S HEALTH CENTER
OF WEST VIRGINIA
3418 Staunton Ave., S.E.
Charleston, WV 25304
(304) 344-9834

NATIONAL FEMINIST, LEGAL AND PUBLIC POLICY ORGANIZATIONS

The following national organizations are committed to keeping abortion safe and legal. They are invaluable resources, providing accurate, in-depth information at the national, state and community level.

ABORTION RIGHTS
MOBILIZATION (ARM)
Abortion advocacy especially on legal issues
Lawrence Lader
51 Fifth Ave.
New York, NY 10003
(212) 255-0682

CATHOLICS FOR
A FREE CHOICE
Provides education on abortion and family planning with an activist network in 55 communities
1436 U St., NW. #301
Washington, DC 20009
(202) 986-6093

CENTER FOR
CONSTITUTIONAL RIGHTS
Legal advocacy for constitutional rights
666 Broadway
New York, NY 10012
(212) 614-6464

CENTER FOR POPULATION
OPTIONS
Public policy organization
1025 Vermont Ave., N.W.
Washington, DC 20009
(202) 347-5700

CENTER FOR
REPRODUCTIVE LAW
AND POLICY
Legal advocacy for reproductive rights
120 Wall St.,
New York, NY 10005
(212) 514-5534

CIVIL LIBERTIES AND
PUBLIC POLICY PROGRAM
Hampshire College
Amherst MA 01002
(413) 549-4600

FEDERATION OF FEMINIST
WOMEN'S HEALTH CENTERS
3701 J St., #201
Sacramento, CA 95816
(916) 451-0621

FEMINIST MAJORITY
FOUNDATION
186 South St.
Boston, MA 02111
(617) 695-9688

FUND FOR THE
FEMINIST MAJORITY
Feminist research and activist organization dedicated to empowering women in all sectors of society
1600 Wilson Blvd., #704
Arlington, VA 22209
(703) 522-2214

FUND FOR THE
FEMINIST MAJORITY
8105 W. 3rd St., #1
Los Angeles CA 90048
(213) 651-0495

HEALTH POLICY ADVISORY
CENTER (HEALTH/PAC)
**A public interest center advo-
cating appropriate and accessible health care for all**
47 W. 14th St., #300
New York NY 10011
(212) 627-1847

MADRE
**A multi-cultural, multi-racial
coalition of 23,000 women in
Central America and the
Middle East**
121 W. 27th St. #301
New York, NY 10001
(212) 627-0444

NATIONAL ABORTION RIGHTS
ACTION LEAGUE (NARAL)
**Abortion rights advocacy
organization**
1101 14th St., N.W.
Washington, DC 20005
(202) 667-5881
(800) 408-4600

NATIONAL BLACK WOMEN'S
HEALTH PROJECT
1237 Ralph David Abernathy
Dr., S.E.
Atlanta, GA 30310
(404) 758-9590

NATIONAL BLACK WOMEN'S
HEALTH PROJECT
Policy/Education Office
1615 M St., N.W., #230
Washington, DC 20036
(202) 835-0117

NATIONAL ORGANIZATION
FOR WOMEN (NOW)
600 chapters nationwide
1000 16th St., N.W.
Washington, DC 20036
(202) 331-0066

NATIONAL WOMEN'S HEALTH
NETWORK ✿
1326 G St., N.W.
Washington, DC 20005
(202) 347-1140

THE OVERGROUND RAILROAD
**Chapters in 40 states,
referrals, transportation
and housing for women
who must travel to obtain
abortions**
P.O. Box 79
Skippack PA 19474
(800) 726-1468 (for abortion
information)

PLANNED PARENTHOOD
FEDERATION OF AMERICA,
INC.
**169 affiliates in U.S.,
900 family planning clinics,
55 of which do abortions**
810 2nd Ave.
New York, NY 10021
(212) 541-7800

THE POPULATION COUNCIL
**Research and public policy
organization**
One Dag Hammarskjold Plaza
New York, NY 10017
(212) 644-1300

POPULATION CRISIS
COMMITTEE
Public policy organization
1120 19th St., N.W., #550
Washington, DC 20036
(202) 659-1833

RELIGIOUS COALITION FOR
ABORTION RIGHTS (RCAR)
**25 local affiliates, educates
and advocates for public
policy following the principles
of the *Roe* decision**
100 Maryland Ave., N.E., #307
Washington, DC 20002
(202) 543-7032

REPRODUCTIVE HEALTH
TECHNOLOGIES PROJECT
**Task force formed to
promote public education
about new reproductive
technologies such as
RU-486**
1601 Connecticut Ave., N.W.
#801
Washington, DC 20009
(202) 328-2200

FINANCIAL ASSISTANCE AND LOAN FUNDS

The following organizations provide direct financial assistance or low- or no-interest loans for abortions. Some may also provide transportation assistance, and information on Medicaid eligibility and how to obtain a judicial bypass if parental notification is required.*

ABORTION RIGHTS FUND OF
WESTERN MASSACHUSETTS
**Provides interest-free loans to
women who need abortions**
P.O. Box 732
Hadley, MA 01035
(413) 582-3532

CHICAGO ABORTION FUND
**Loans/grants available
for young teens and women
without financial resources**
Stacy Haugland
P.O. Box 578307
Chicago IL 60613
(312) 248-4541

COUNCIL ON ABORTION
RIGHTS EDUCATION (CARE)
**Most recipients are women of
color who reside in
Minnasota, Wisconsin, North
Dakota, South Dakota, Illinois
and Iowa, but the Council is
committed to helping "any
woman, anywhere."**
3255 Hennepin Ave. #227
Minneapolis MN 55408
(612) 827-5827

FREEDOM FUND
**Funding for teens less than
12 weeks pregnant who live
in Colorado, with priority
given to Denver area**
Margie Wullschleger
1616 17th St., #472
Denver, CO 80202
(303) 628-5472

---

*Special thanks to Sabrae Jenkins of the Women of Color Partnership Program, Washington, D.C., 202-543-9060, who compiled this list.

GREATER PHILADELPHIA
WOMEN'S FUND
**Loans and assistance for
women with low incomes who
are residents of the greater
Philadelphia area**
Shawn Tooey
1218 Chestnut St., #1007
Philadelphia PA 19107
(215) 923-4046

HERSHEY ABORTION
ASSISTANCE FUND
**Direct financial assistance
and abortion referrals.
Not limited to Minnesota
residents.**
Kelly Lynch
Pro-Choice Resources
3255 Hennepin Ave. S., #255
Minneapolis MN 55408
(612) 825-9122

LAST RESORT FUND
**Abortion assistance for
reported cases of rape and
incest, documented grossfetal
deformity, danger to health of
mother, or women diagnosed
with HIV or AIDS. Available to
residents of Colorado, New
Mexico,Wyoming, or perhaps
other states.**
Sylvia Clark
Planned Parenthood
of Denver
2030 20th Ave.
Denver CO 80205
(303) 321-2458

NORTHERN VIRGINIA
JUSTICE FUND
**Loan assistance for Medicaid
eligible women in Northern
Virgina**
Pat Kibler
Planned Parenthood of
Northern Virginia
5622 Columbia Pike, #303
Falls Church, VA 20910
(703) 820-3335

PLANNED PARENTHOOD OF
METROPOLITAN WASHINGTON
**Reduced or deferred
payment for clients who are
in need: "No one will be
turned away."**
1180 16th St., N.W.
Washington, DC 20036
(202) 347-8500

PLANNED PARENTHOOD OF
SOUTHEAST TEXAS JUSTICE
FUND
**Loan assistance based
on need for women in
Southeast Texas**
Virginia Miller
Planned Parenthood
of Southeast Texas
3601 Fanin
Houston, TX 77004
(713) 522-6240

JIM WIMBERLY
LOAN FUND
**Direct abortion referrals and
loan assistance or funds for
Medicaid-eligible women
living in or around Austin.**
Nancy Sasaki
Planned Parenthood
of Austin
1290 Rosewood Ave.
Austin, TX 78702
(512) 472-0868

WOMEN IN NEED FUND
Women who qualify for Title X, Medicaid or Medicare. Funding extends outside of Georgia.
Ava Bowden
Atlanta Feminist Women's
Health Center
1575 Northside Dr.,
Bldg. 100
Atlanta GA 30319
(404) 351-7105

THE NATIONAL ABORTION FEDERATION, 800-543-6240, may have information on other funds and assistance programs.

INTERNATIONAL WOMEN'S HEALTH PROJECTS AND INFORMATION CLEARINGHOUSES

This list of international women's health projects and resource centers includes organizations that have a global focus and a commitment to women's health concerns. These groups provide general information on a wide range of women's health issues.*

AUSTRALIA

HEALTHSHARING WOMEN
318 Little Bourke St.
Melbourne, Australia 3000

WOMEN'S HEALTH
INFORMATION RESOURCE
COLLECTIVE, INC.
P.O. Box 187
N. Carlton, Victoria
Australia 3054

BANGLADESH

BANGLADESH WOMEN'S
HEALTH COALITION
House 46-A, Dhanmondi Rd.
Dhaka 1205, Bangladesh

BRAZIL

SOS CORPO
Rua do Hospicio
859-4 Oandar
Boa Vista
Recife, Brazil 50050

* Special thanks to the Boston Women's Health Book Collective and Lorraine Rothman and Shauna Heckert for contributions to this list.

CANADA

HEALTHSHARING,
Women Healthsharing
14 Skey Ln.
Toronto, Ontario M6J 3S4,
Canada

MONTREAL HEALTH PRESS,
INC.
C.P. 1000
Station Place du Parc
Montreal, Quebec, Canada H2W
2N1

GERMANY

FEMINISTISCHES FRAUEN-
GESUNDHEITS ZENTRUM E.V.
Bamberger Str. 51
1000 Berlin 30,
Germany

INDIA

RESEARCH UNIT ON WOMEN'S
STUDIES at SNDT Women's
University
Juhu Campus
Bombay, India 400-049

IRELAND

THE DUBLIN WELL WOMAN
CENTER
73 Lower Leeson St.
Dublin 2, Ireland

MALAYSIA

WOMEN'S DEVELOPMENT
PROGRAM
Asian and Pacific Development
Center
P.O. Box 12224
50770 Kuala Lampur
Malaysia

MEXICO

COMUNICACION
INTERCAMBIO Y DESARROLO
HUMANO EN AMERICA LATINA
(CIDHAL)
Apdo 579
Cuernavaca, Morelos,
Mexico

NETHERLANDS

STIMEZO, INTERNATIONAL
Pieterstraatt 11
3512 JT Utrecht
The Netherlands

WOMEN'S GLOBAL NETWORK
FOR REPRODUCTIVE RIGHTS
(WGNRR)
NZ Voorburgwal 32
1012RZ, Amsterdam,
The Netherlands

NICARAGUA

AMALIE
Reparto San Juan
Entrada Principal,
2 1/2 Cuandras al Sur
Managua, Nicaragua

PHILIPPINES

ISIS INTERNATIONAL
85-A East Maya St.
Philamlife Homes
Quezon City 0000, Philippines

WOMANHEALTH PHILLIPINES
125B Gonzales St.
Loyola Heights
Quezon City 1108, Philippines

SPAIN

BELEN NOQUIEREZ
Espacio de Salud Para Mujeres
Avda Alfonso XIII, 118

COLECTIVO DE SALUD
SPECULUM
Herrera el Viejo No. 6
41001 Seville, Spain

JUSTA Montero
Concha Delgado
Comision Pro Derecho al Aborto
Barquillo 44 21ZQ
28004 Madrid, Spain

SWITZERLAND

ISIS-WICCE
3 Chemin des Campanules
1291 Aire
Geneva, Switzerland

UNITED KINGDOM

WOMEN'S HEALTH AND
REPRODUCTIVE RIGHTS
INFORMATION CENTRE
52 Featherstone St.
London EC1Y 8RT
England

CHAPTER THREE

The Best Available Abortion Care

AFTER YOU have made up your mind to terminate a pregnancy and know where to find a reputable clinic or qualified doctor, you may still be apprehensive about the quality of care you will receive once you get there. If you live in a metropolitan area and don't have to travel to get an abortion, you might have difficulty in evaluating the claims of competing clinics. You may also be confused by myths and misinformation about abortion spread by anti-abortion groups. Getting a legal abortion requires that you be informed in order to make the right choices. And if you are faced with getting an illegal abortion, being well-informed may help you avoid a life-threatening situation.

To help make the search for safe abortion care easier, this chapter exposes common myths about abortion, describes what we believe to be a high standard of abortion care, and provides information that can help you get the safest abortion possible.

MYTHS AND FACTS ABOUT ABORTION

After abortion became legal, the topic was discussed openly and many old myths and folk tales that had evolved in the absence of reliable scientific information began to fade into the past. But in the past few years, the anti-abortion movement has resurrected these myths— and dreamed up new ones—in efforts to dissuade women from having abortions. Here are the myths and the facts.

MYTH: Abortion is dangerous.

FACT: When done by an experienced practitioner, early termination suction abortion is one of the safest of all medical procedures.[1] In suction procedures, major complications are extremely rare, occurring less than 1% of the time when the abortion is done by a skilled practitioner. Less skilled practitioners may have slightly higher complication rates. In later abortion, the complication rate increases, but this procedure is still very safe when compared to other surgical procedures. *One salient fact that the anti-abortion movement cannot afford to acknowledge is that childbirth is 11 times more dangerous than early termination abortion.* [2]

MYTH: Many women who have abortions suffer from a "post-abortion syndrome," including depression, anger, grief, nightmares, and feeling exploited and dehumanized.

FACT: Anti-abortion activists have dredged up outdated and poorly done psychological studies from when abortion was still illegal in attempts to support this myth, but an exhaustively researched study of abortion by Dr. C. Everett Koop, Surgeon General during the Reagan administration, found no evidence for the existence of such a syndrome.[3] *Depression among women after childbirth, however, is well documented.*

MYTH: Abortion is unavailable after about 16 weeks of pregnancy.

FACT: In many states, abortion remains legal to 22 or 24 weeks from the last menstrual period, and in a few places to 26 weeks. (For information on how to find practitioners who do abortions after 16 weeks, see "The NAF Hotline," page 9).

MYTH: Several abortions may make it difficult to carry future pregnancies to term.

FACT: Complications from *illegal* abortions sometimes made it difficult for women to carry subsequent pregnancies successfully, but there is no medical evidence that this is true for early abortions, or for most later abortions, when they are done by trained personnel.

Myth: Abortions may cause complications in later deliveries.

FACT: Ninety percent of abortions are done in the first trimester, and complications are exceedingly rare. While the rate of complications increases during the second trimester, with appropriate medical treatment these *rarely* affect a woman's ability to carry subsequent pregnancies to term.

MYTH: Abortion causes infertility.

FACT: Infertility was a common result of illegal abortions, when an infection or perforation often occurred, but it is almost unheard of today when skilled practitioners use sterile procedures and flexible instruments.

PREGNANCY DIAGNOSIS

If you suspect you are pregnant—whether or not you want to terminate the pregnancy—you should get a pregnancy test as soon as possible so that you can begin searching for an abortion provider, or see a doctor or midwife to begin pre-natal care. Today, home pregnancy tests costing between $15 and $25 are available in most pharmacies, and these tests are generally accurate on or about the first day of your expected period, or about 14 days after conception. However, home pregnancy tests are not considered to be a definitive diagnosis, so your clinic or doctor will do another chemical pregnancy test, as well as a bi-manual pelvic examination, which, in most cases, is considered sufficient to diagnose pregnancy. If a doctor is not sure how far pregnant you are, he or she may order a sonogram (see page 75) and blood pregnancy test, called a Beta HCG (human chorionic gonadotropin, the hormone of pregnancy), test which is accurate seven to 10 days after conception.

ESTIMATING THE LAST NORMAL MENSTRUAL PERIOD (LNMP)

Most women know when they had their last period and many can accurately determine that they are pregnant by observing subjective signs, such as sore breasts, bloating, changes in appetite, fatigue, and a missed period (see *Signs of Pregnancy*, page 140). **Sometimes, however, one or more of the following occurrences can make the signs of pregnancy difficult to interpret:**

➡ Even though fertilization has occurred, some women have a "false" menstrual period, which may be lighter or shorter than normal. If a false period is suspected, then the last "normal" period should be used to calculate the length of pregnancy.

➡ Sometimes spotting or bleeding, which may be mistaken for a period, is actually a sign of an impending miscarriage or a tubal pregnancy.

➡ Some women don't keep track of their periods, but may have some general idea of how often they get them. If periods come irregularly, it is often difficult for a woman to know when to expect her next period. In this case, the size of the uterus, as measured by the doctor in a bi-manual pelvic exam, is essential in determining gestational age.

BIRTH CONTROL PILL
MAY CLOUD THE ISSUE

If you got pregnant while taking birth control pills, estimating when you got pregnant may be more difficult because:

➡ women who take birth control pills often do not see themselves at risk for pregnancy, especially if they take their pills conscientiously; therefore, some women may not suspect that they are pregnant until they have missed more than one period.

➡ signs of pregnancy are similar to the side effects of the pill, especially bloating and breast tenderness, weight gain, and changes in appetite.

➡ some women have no bleeding at all while on the pill, and thus do not have a missed period as a marker of pregnancy.

➡ normal periods may not resume immediately after pill discontinuation, and may thus make pregnancy more difficult to detect.

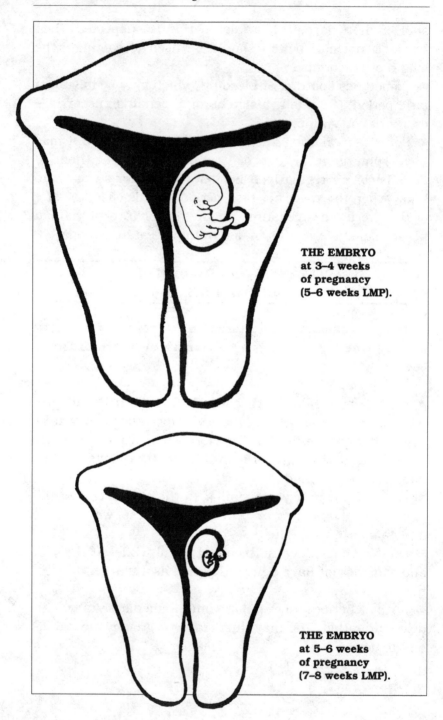

**THE EMBRYO
at 3–4 weeks
of pregnancy
(5–6 weeks LMP).**

**THE EMBRYO
at 5–6 weeks
of pregnancy
(7–8 weeks LMP).**

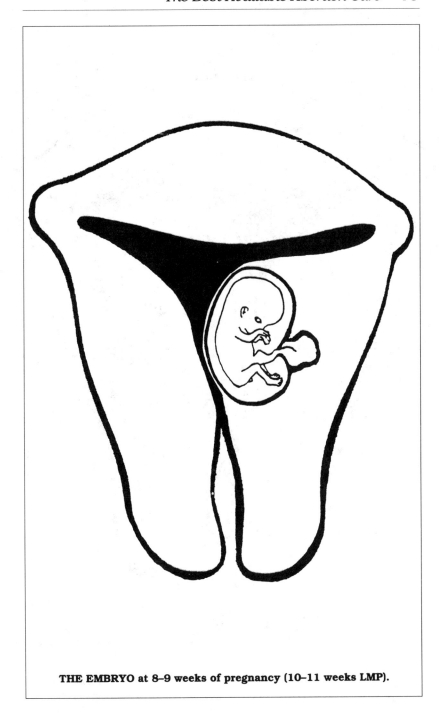

THE EMBRYO at 8–9 weeks of pregnancy (10–11 weeks LMP).

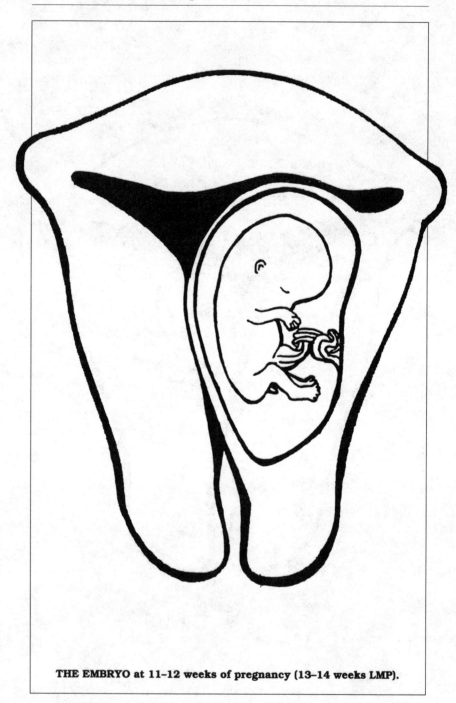

THE EMBRYO at 11–12 weeks of pregnancy (13–14 weeks LMP).

SONOGRAMS

A sonogram provides an X-ray-like picture made with high frequency sound waves, called *ultrasound,* instead of radiation. The sound waves bounce off organs and structures of different density and are transformed electronically into a picture of the inside of the uterus. In early pregnancy, sonograms are not routinely used, but may be helpful in estimating gestational age for women who are unsure of when they got pregnant, or for young women whose menstrual cycles are irregular.

If you are pretty sure that your pregnancy is well under 13 weeks from your last period, and a clinic says that you need a sonogram, it is perfectly appropriate to ask the reason, especially if there is an additional charge. If you are told that everyone gets a sonogram, you can be relatively certain that you, or your insurance company, is being charged for an unnecessary procedure. In the second trimester, sonograms are routinely used to get an accurate picture of gestational age, in order to be sure that you are not over the limit beyond which the doctor is unable to do the procedure.

Uterine sonograms generally work best if a woman has a full bladder (to make it easier to distinguish from the uterus), so you will be asked to drink several glasses of water and wait 20 to 30 minutes for your bladder to fill. This can be uncomfortable for pregnant women, so some clinics don't require that the bladder be totally full. Then a technician will spread some lubricant over your abdomen and pass a sensor over the area, making a picture of the interior of your uterus.

INFORMATIONAL COUNSELING

Ideally, every woman who seeks an abortion should have access to informative, supportive counseling that acquaints her with her options, describes the risks and benefits of each, and provides clear instructions on what to look for immediately after the procedure, as well as what to expect in the next few weeks until she gets a normal period. This *informational counseling* is designed to answer questions that typically arise concerning the abortion procedure; it is a standard part of most clinic routines but may or may not be available in doctors' offices. Women who have had abortions often say that knowing exactly what was going to happen during the procedure calmed anxieties and helped them feel more in control.

PSYCHOLOGICAL COUNSELING

By the time most women arrive at a clinic, they have made up their minds to terminate their pregnancies, and do not want or need psychological counseling. Yet some women do feel ambivalent about abortion, or about their decision, and may need help in resolving their feelings before the procedure, and perhaps afterward.

If you have conflicts or questions about abortion, and don't have the benefit of supportive counseling, it might be wise to try to find a counselor, family member, or friend who will help you think things through. It might be especially helpful to try to visualize your life in a year if 1) you have an abortion, or 2) you continue your pregnancy. It might also be useful to assess how dependable your partner will be in sharing in the upbringing of a child. And you might also want to compare the costs of an abortion with those of childbirth, and calculate the outlay for baby clothes, diapers, medical expenses and other items during the first year.

**CONCERNS WOMEN MAY HAVE
BEFORE AN ABORTION**

➡ Not wanting to face the fact that pregnancy occurred.

➡ Feeling guilty/irresponsible/stupid for having gotten pregnant.

➡ Fearing for future infertility after an abortion.

➡ Fearing pain or complications during the abortion procedure.

➡ Feeling sad or upset that personal or financial situation does not permit the birth of a child.

➡ Feeling that abortion is wrong.

➡ Fearing that a relationship will end if you have an abortion or if you don't have one.

➡ Having conflicts with partner or husband over the decision to have an abortion.

HOW WOMEN FEEL AFTER AN ABORTION

There is no one way to feel after an abortion. Some women may feel troubled or depressed, but these feelings are not caused, as abortion foes have suggested, by severe hormonal changes. Contrary to popular belief, few women actually regret their decisions to have an abortion. Some women do regret that circumstances in their lives—their age, financial circumstances, career obligations or problems with their partners—make it difficult at the moment to have a child. As Nora, the young mother of a two-year-old, who decided to have an abortion rather than have a second child, told her counselor, "This is my decision, but it is not my choice."

What the majority of women feel after an abortion is *relief and happiness*[4]—relief that the procedure wasn't as bad as they had imagined it would be, and happiness that they don't have to make a major life decision suddenly, just because they forgot to take a pill, use a condom or cervical cap, or because they were forced or persuaded to have sex when they didn't want to.

In an essay in *The New York Times* "Hers" column,[5] author Barbara Ehrenreich described her feelings after an abortion:

> *Quite apart from blowing up clinics and terrorizing patients, the anti-abortion movement can take credit for a more subtle and lasting kind of damage: It has succeeded in getting even pro-choice people to think of abortion as a "moral dilemma," an "agonizing decision" and related code phrases for something murky and compromising, like the traffic in infant formula mix. In liberal circles, it has become unstylish to discuss abortion without using words like "complex," "painful" and the rest of the mealy-mouthed vocabulary of evasion. Regrets are also fashionable, and one otherwise feminist author writes recently of mourning, each year following her abortion, the putative birthday of her discarded fetus. I cannot speak for other women, of course, but the one regret I have about my own abortions is that they cost money that might otherwise have been spent on something more pleasurable, like taking the kids to movies and theme parks....*

Whatever women feel about abortion, they have a right to have those feelings taken seriously, and abortion providers have a responsibility to help resolve confusion, ambivalence, or guilt before the procedure is done.

LOCAL VERSUS GENERAL ANESTHESIA

The decision to have general anesthesia is often based on the perception that abortion is a major surgical procedure and is therefore painful, and perhaps scary. However, in most early abortions, the cannula, the straw-like instrument that is inserted into the uterus, is only inside the uterus for two to three minutes, and there is no cutting or scraping of the uterine wall.

The majority of abortion clinics in the United States do early abortions under local anesthesia. ("Local" means "at the site of the procedure," which in this case is the cervix, the neck of the uterus that protrudes into the vagina.) This involves an injection of a novacaine-type drug directly into the cervix. Some women actually find the injection the most uncomfortable part of procedure, but the discomfort only lasts as long as it takes to give the injection—about 15 to 20 seconds. Actually, "local anesthesia" is something of a misnomer. A "local" does make dilation of the cervical canal, which is pretty minimal in an early abortion, easier, but it does nothing to diminish the cramping that results as the uterus is emptied and contracts back to its pre-pregnancy size.

Since an early abortion takes only two or three minutes, it is unnecessary in most cases to use general anesthesia, although it is often offered as an option. However, in some hospitals, general anesthesia may be the only option, even though most of the risks associated with most abortions have to do with general anesthesia.

Some women may feel such guilt or shame about needing an abortion they want to be "knocked out" so that they won't know what's happening during the procedure and therefore aren't "responsible." But general anesthesia has some distinct disadvantages. When you are unconscious, a doctor has the freedom to use larger instruments, especially a curette, and may work faster and less gently—factors thought to contribute to a higher incidence of complications, particularly uterine perforation and hemorrhage. In addition, there is the small, but very real, risk of death associated with general anesthesia for any surgical procedure—about 1 in 10,000—and this includes abortion. Most deaths from abortion are anesthesia-related.

Under local anesthesia, you are conscious throughout the procedure and can monitor the practitioner's behavior and conversation with assistants, and you can tell him or her how you are feeling, especially if you feel unusual pain or discomfort. You can also make sure that you are treated respectfully at all times.

Cheryl, a counselor in an abortion clinic in San Diego, California, describes the differences in women's recovery from local and general anesthesia:

> With local anesthesia, some women feel little or no aftereffects and go right back to work, go to lunch with a friend, or go dancing that night. Others, however, just want to take it easy for the rest of the day. On the other hand, women who have general anesthesia wake up groggy and nauseous. Some types of general anesthesia also cause scary dreams, and women sometimes wake up crying. It's not unusual for women to stay in recovery for an hour or more after having general anesthesia, and some say they don't feel well for one to two days. Some women also report having disturbing feelings that may stem from not knowing what happened to them while they were unconscious.

ABORTION TERMINOLOGY

FIRST TRIMESTER ABORTION: An abortion done up to 11 weeks gestation or 13 weeks from the last normal menstrual period (LNMP).

SECOND TRIMESTER ABORTION: An abortion done after 11 weeks gestation or 13 weeks LNMP, sometimes referred to as a "later abortion."

EARLY TERMINATION SUCTION ABORTION: The uterine contents are evacuated by means of suction, using flexible plastic cannulas with a minimum of cervical dilation. A

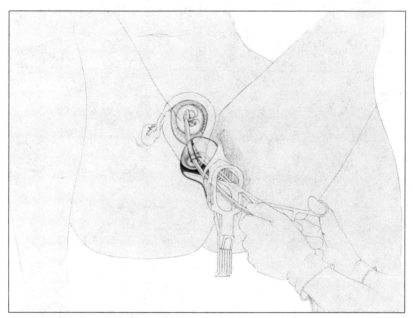

DURING AN EARLY termination suction abortion, the cannula, held in the doctor's left hand, is inserted through the cervical canal into the uterus. The uterine contents are suctioned out through the cannula. With the right hand, the doctor is holding a tenaculum, a long tweezer-like clamp that helps stabilize the cervix during the procedure.

curette is only used if there is a compelling reason. This procedure is *twice as safe* as the old-fashioned D&C.

SUCTION CURETTAGE: A combination of suction abortion and a D&C.

DILATION & CURETTAGE (D&C): An abortion technique in which the cervix is dilated with graduated metal rods, the uterine wall is scraped with a curette, and tissue or fetal parts are removed with forceps. Suction may or may not be used as an adjunct.

DILATION & EVACUATION (D&E): The preferred later abortion procedure, which employs laminaria and/or large metal dilators, a curette, forceps, and suction.

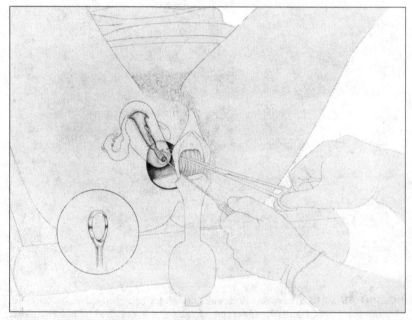

ALTHOUGH THE USE of a curette is usually unnecessary, some doctors still use one after suctioning out the uterine contents. The inset shows the head of the curette. In this illustration, the doctor is using a weighted metal speculum. Many clinics now use disposable plastic speculums, which women generally find less uncomfortable.

CANNULA: A flexible plastic straw-like instrument that is inserted into the uterus through which the uterine contents are suctioned out. Cannulas range in size from 4mm, which is extremely soft and flexible, to the rigid 16mm size.

CURETTE: A razor-sharp, spoon-like metal instrument used to scrape pregnancy tissue from the uterine wall in the D&C procedure. Curettes are not necessary in most first trimester abortions.

DILATORS: Graduated metal rods that are inserted into the cervical canal to widen it enough to accommodate a cannula.

FORCEPS: A tong-like instrument used in later second trimester abortions to remove fetal parts.

LAMINARIA: Sticks of compressed seaweed about the size of kitchen matches, which expand gradually when inserted into the cervix, stretching the opening to accommodate instruments and allowing for the removal of fetal parts. One or more sticks may be inserted at a time, and are removed just prior to the abortion. Laminaria are routinely used to provide a safer, gentler way to dilate the cervix in second trimester abortions than metal dilators, but can also reduce the discomfort of dilation in first trimester procedures as well.

SPECULUM: A plastic or metal duck-billed instrument used to spread the walls of the vagina to provide a view of, and access to, the cervix.

TENACULUM: A long-handled tweezer-like instrument with pincers on the end used to grasp and stabilize the cervix during an abortion.

THE EXPERIENCE OF ABORTION

Sophia, a 26-year-old dental assistant, recently got an abortion at a women's clinic in southern California:

I had one abortion when I was 18, and it was a pretty awful experience. Although the clinic was nice enough, there was a sort of abortion-mill atmosphere, and they gave me general anesthesia, which made me feel lousy for a couple of days. This time I decided not to have general anesthesia, but I was a little nervous about being awake during the abortion. I went to the clinic at 11:00 on a Saturday morning, and was with four other women who were also getting abortions. Our counselor, Jean, stayed with us the whole time. First she helped us fill out our forms. We all gave urine samples, and a nurse took our blood pressure, drew some blood and did a finger prick to test for anemia. Then Jean told us what was going to happen during the abortion, how we would probably feel during the procedure, and what to look for afterward. She said the more relaxed we were, the easier it would be, and offered us a mild tranquilizer. I decided I should get all the help I could, and took it. It was very mild and I didn't feel much different at all. Jean also asked if anyone felt uncomfortable about the decision to have an abortion and said if we did, we could speak to a counselor individually. One woman in the group did see the counselor and later said it helped her to feel more sure about her decision.

When my turn came, Jean took me into one of the procedure rooms and told me to undress from the waist down and sit on the exam table. I was very happy that she was going to stay with me during the abortion, so I wouldn't have to face some strange doctor alone. Soon the doctor came in and Jean introduced us, and that made me feel good too. I felt like we were just a little more equal. Then Jean had me lie down on the table and helped me put my feet in the stirrups. The doctor told me he was going to do a pelvic exam to feel the size of my uterus, and after he did it, said he thought I was about eight weeks from my last period. Jean explained that he meant I was actually about six weeks pregnant, which was about what I had figured out.

The doctor put a speculum in place and told me he was going to swab my vagina with iodine to decrease the chance of infection. That felt a little cold but not bad. Then he said he was going to attach a "stabilizer" to my cervix in order to give the injection of anesthetic, and that I might feel a pinch or some slight cramps. I guess I felt both, but it was a little hard to separate the sensations. The doctor told me he was going to give me the injection of anesthetic in my cervix, and that I might feel a sting and some cramping. I felt a sharp sting, and kind of an achy pressure, and some definite cramps. While we were waiting a minute for the anesthetic to take effect, Jean asked me if I usually have strong cramps during my period—which I do—and she said that women who have heavy menstrual cramps sometimes have heavier cramps during an abortion. She reminded me that the abortion itself would only take about two or three minutes, and that the more relaxed I was, the less uncomfortable the procedure would be. By now about one minute had passed, and the assistant handed the doctor the cannula, which was attached to a tube that ran into a jar. The jar was attached to a machine that Jean called an aspirator. The doctor told me that he was going to insert the cannula into my cervical canal, and that I might feel some more cramping, especially when the cannula passed the "inner os," the band of muscle that keeps the interior of the uterus separated from the cervical canal.

Jean took my hand and told me to take a few deep breaths and to count to 10 as I let them out. My uterus was starting to rebel. I tried to think of something else. "Okay, the cannula is in, and the suction is going to be turned on," she said. I heard a loud hum and I could tell that the doctor was moving the cannula. The cramps were pretty strong now, and my thighs were beginning to ache. Maybe I was starting to sweat and to make some noises, because Jane said, "Sophia, look at

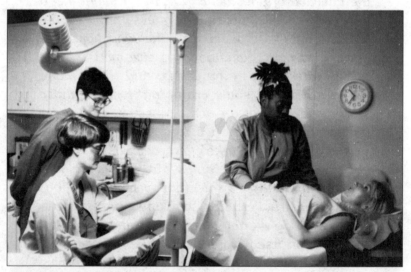

THIS PHOTOGRAPH SHOWS an abortion at the Atlanta Feminist Women's Health Center. The doctor is seated on the left, and her assistant is standing behind her. A counselor, standing on the right, is with the woman throughout the abortion procedure.

me." I opened my eyes, and instead of seeing stars, I saw her face. "How are you feeling?" she asked. "Well, if you really want to know, I'd rather be roller-skating," I said. "Well, you will be in just a few minutes," she replied. She asked the doctor how much longer before he finished. He said, "About one minute or less." "Okay," Jean said. "This is the countdown. Let me know if you feel funny in any way." Suddenly the cramps got stronger, and I felt a sharp pinching sensation in my uterus. I hoped I would never have a period like this. "Thirty seconds," Jean said. "Take three deep breaths, let them out slowly, and it will be over." But before I got to three, the doctor said, "You can relax. It's all over." "I am *relaxed!*" I said, but since it was hardly true, we all burst out laughing. Jean wiped my forehead with a cool cloth, and said that I should lie there for a few minutes until I felt like moving. She also suggested that I pull my knees up to my chest and then stretch them out to try to relieve some of the muscle tension. The pinching sensation was gone, and the cramps were becoming tolerable. In about three or four minutes, Jean helped me sit up, and since I felt okay, she handed my clothes to me and I got dressed. I really was a little shaky, so I lay down in the after-care room for about 10 or 15 minutes, then the counselor took my blood pressure and asked about my cramps. By now they felt like a regular period. Another counselor gave me some aftercare information and told me to call a special number if anything unusual occurred. In all, I was in the clinic about two and one-half hours. That night my boyfriend and I went to a movie and then drove to the beach. I felt completely recovered.

Sophia's experience is fairly typical of early termination suction abortions. Nothing unusual occurred. Sensations of cramping and pain are often heightened if a woman is anxious or frightened; the more relaxed she is, the less uncomfortable she will be during an abortion. Supportive advocacy during the procedure can relieve tension and anxiety.

UNUSUAL PHYSICAL REACTIONS DURING AN ABORTION

About 2% of women experience unusual—but normal—reactions during the procedure, such as hyperventilation, fainting, or vaso-vagal response. **These reactions are not serious in any way, but can be frightening if women are unprepared for them.**

HYPERVENTILATION: Stress or tension can sometimes result in hyperventilation: rapid, shallow breathing caused by an imbalance in blood carbon dioxide. If hyperventilation occurs, you may experience lightheadedness, faintness, and even panic, and may have a hard time regaining control over your breathing. In extreme cases, women may actually faint.

If you begin to hyperventilate, there are several simple techniques you can use to control breathing and restore the balance of oxygen and carbon dioxide in the bloodstream, including taking deep, measured breaths, closing one nostril with a finger while breathing through the other nostril, and breathing into a paper (not a plastic) bag for a few minutes. All of these maneuvers can help restore the oxygen/carbon dioxide balance in your bloodstream.

FAINTING: Fainting, the temporary loss of consciousness, is caused by decreased blood flow to the brain, and is usually preceded by nausea, stomach distress, sweating and pallor. During an abortion, fainting is usually associated with a vaso-vagal response (see below). If you do faint, you will probably recover in about 30 seconds. Routine first-aid techniques such as elevating your feet and placing your head lower than your chest can help avoid fainting. Ammonia capsules are generally unnecessary, but may speed recovery.

VASO-VAGAL RESPONSE: Occasionally during an abortion, most commonly near the end, the vagus, the major nerve that runs down each leg, can be stimulated, resulting in a dramatic, but benign physical reaction. Your skin may feel cool, clammy, or sweaty, and you may become very pale. Pulse and blood pressure may be lowered, and you may feel faint, dizzy, or nauseous, especially if you try to stand or sit up, and, because of muscle tension, your limbs may go stiff. The vagal response can be uncomfortable, but it is of short duration and will pass on its own. Standard first aid techniques for fainting are generally sufficient for revival. If choking or vomiting does occur, whether associated with a vagal response or not, the nurse or counselor needs to make sure you are lying down, and that your head is to the side to prevent choking.

SECOND TRIMESTER ABORTION

The procedure for second trimester abortions, which by definition are those done between 13 and 26 weeks from the last menstrual period, is essentially the same as for first trimester abortion procedures, but with some variation.

The standard technique used for second trimester abortions is *dilation and evacuation* (D&E). This procedure is similar to a suction curettage procedure, although larger instruments are used, and most of the dilation is done before the procedure begins with *laminaria*, sticks of compressed seaweed about the size of large kitchen matches. (*Dilapan* is a new synthetic laminaria.) Overnight, the laminaria will absorb cervical secretions and expand, dilating the cervix slowly and gently. Most women experience mild cramping from the laminaria, although some have fairly strong cramps. Occasionally, the laminaria will actually precipitate a miscarriage, so if you are having strong cramps that come in waves, call your practitioner. He or she can evaluate your situation and tell you what to do. Depending on how far pregnant you are, you may have laminaria inserted once or twice. In each session, from five to 10 sticks will be inserted and left in place from about six hours to overnight.

In abortions over 20 weeks, many clinics administer an injection of *Digoxin*, a drug normally given as an antidote to toxicity from digitalis. A small amount of this drug stops the fetal heartbeat, makes the abortion easier, and avoids the prospect of delivering a live, but severely damaged fetus.

Most women having D&Es, especially those who are more than 20 weeks pregnant, are required to have gen-

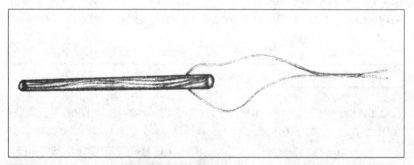

IN SECOND, AND sometimes in first trimester abortions as well, sticks of compressed seaweed, called laminaria, are inserted into the cervical canal. Over a period of six to eight hours, or overnight, the seaweed expands, gently dilating the cervical canal. In late second trimester abortions, up to ten sticks may be inserted at a time. (This laminaria stick is shown actual size).

eral anesthesia because the longer second trimester abortion would otherwise be quite painful. In the D&E procedure, which usually takes from five to 15 minutes, the doctor removes the laminaria, then removes the fetal parts with forceps, scrapes the walls of the uterus with a curette, and completes the procedure by evacuating blood and remaining bits of tissue with suction.

Recovery from a second trimester abortion is somewhat dependent on how far pregnant a woman was and on the type of anesthetic used. Some clinics use narcotics such as *fentanyl citrate* (Sublimaze), given intravenously, as opposed to stronger morphine derivatives. Milder analgesics such as fentanyl put you under but not *out*, and recovery is much quicker.

After a second trimester abortion, women usually remain at the clinic from 45 minutes to two hours. Many clinics do second trimester procedures on Fridays so that women have the weekend to recover. According to the reports of several clinic directors, women who work are generally able to return to work on Monday.

Because of the complex factors that usually cause women to seek later abortions, a D&E is very often a more difficult experience emotionally. These factors include denial of pregnancy, the failure to recognize the signs of pregnancy, mistaking signs of pregnancy for some other conditions, ambivalence about terminating the pregnancy, difficulties in obtaining money, lack of access to abortion facilities, relationship difficulties, conflicts about the abortion, and parental notification requirements. All of these difficulties can increase stress and amplify—sometimes disproportionately—normal fears and tensions about the abortion itself. Clinics that routinely do second trimester abortions have counselors who are experienced in dealing with problems that may arise, and are usually happy to do what they can to make the experience easier for you.

BREAST ENGORGEMENT

One problem that women who have later second trimester abortions often experience is breast engorgement, which can be disconcerting because the breasts can be painful to touch and may actually leak. This engorgement, which can cause significant enlargement, usually takes longer than other signs of pregnancy to dissipate—often from two to three weeks.

In the past, many women were given medications to suppress milk production, but they were ineffective for so many women that this practice has largely been discontinued. Many clinics now advise women to be patient and in the meantime, to bind their breasts with elastic bandages or to wear tight bras, and not to touch or stimulate the breasts, which can prolong engorgement. Aspirin or other mild analgesics may ease pain or discomfort.

RHO-GAM INJECTION FOR WOMEN WHO HAVE RH-NEGATIVE BLOOD

About 10% of the population has RH-negative blood, so if you are RH-negative, the chance that you will get pregnant by a man who has RH-positive blood is not insignificant. If this happens, the blood of the fetus could be RH-positive or RH-negative. If the fetus' blood is RH-positive, then your immune system will manufacture antibodies (protective substances in the blood stream that attack and destroy foreign substances) to RH-positive blood. During the first pregnancy, this usually isn't a problem, but in subsequent pregnancies, if the fetus has RH-positive blood, RH-negative antibodies can cross the placenta and attack fetal cells, causing anemia, jaundice, and liver problems. To counteract this potential problem, all women who have RH-negative blood are given an injection of human RH_0 (D) immune globulin (the most common brand name is RhoGAM). For women who are less than 12 weeks pregnant, clinics generally give a mini-dose (Mini-Gamulin), and give women over 12 weeks a full dose. Generally, there is an extra charge for RhoGAM (about $50) and for Mini-Gam (about $25).

WHAT TO EXPECT AFTER AN ABORTION

After an abortion, both first and second trimester, you can expect some period-like cramping for a few hours or even for a day or two, although some women experience almost no cramping afterward. Most women have some bleeding, ranging from spotting to a period-like flow, which may start and stop, and may even resume again, for up to three weeks afterward. Some women may also pass large clots for a day or so after the procedure. Many clinics provide *methylergonovine maleate* (Methergine) tablets to take home, and advise you to take them if you have strong cramps or are passing large clots. Methergine may make the cramps stronger initially, but it helps the uterus contract, and thus, helps control bleeding.

SIGNS OF A COMPLETE ABORTION

The signs of pregnancy—increased appetite, nausea, bloating, and fatigue—should begin to disappear within a few days after an abortion, but breast enlargement may take one to two weeks to disappear entirely. If you feel like you still might be pregnant and want some reassurance, an over-the-counter pregnancy test should become negative one to three weeks after the abortion. Bleeding generally tapers off, but may stop and start again, or you may spot off and on; these patterns can persist for up to three weeks. When you go for your follow-up appointment, your practitioner will do a bi-manual pelvic exam to ascertain that the uterus is not tender when touched, and that it is firm and about the size of a walnut shell. A speculum exam should reveal that the cervical opening is closed.

SIGNS OF A PROBLEM

Your practitioner should carefully instruct you to recognize the signs of a problem, and tell you what to do if one arises.

PROBLEM	SIGN	WHAT TO DO
Incomplete abortion	Signs of pregnancy continue for more than 10 days	Call clinic.
Infection	Fever of more than 100.4°F	Call clinic.
Unusual or heavy bleeding	Using more than one menstrual pad per hour	Take Methergine and call clinic if bleeding does not decrease in 2 to 3 hours.
Uterine perforation	Pain in abdomen that continues for more than a few hours	Call clinic.

If you have any of these signs after you are home, it would be wise to call your practitioner at once, report what you are experiencing, and get an evaluation. If your abortion provider is not available, don't hesitate to call your family doctor or go to the nearest emergency room.

SERIOUS ABORTION COMPLICATIONS

Although abortion is a low-risk procedure, occasionally problems such as hemorrhage, uterine perforation, or tubal pregnancy, do arise. If your practitioner is experienced, these problems can often be dealt with in the clinic, and your condition can be monitored by phone after you leave. At other times, it may be safer to transfer you to an emergency care facility. The serious problems that can arise during an abortion are discussed in detail in "What Practitioners Need to Know About Abortion Complications" (See page 221).

BE PREPARED!

As abortion becomes less available, finding adequate abortion care is going to become far more difficult for many women. You may not want to know all the details of what an abortion entails, and you may be inclined to just pick up the phone, make one call, and check out mentally until it's all over. However, when you are lying on an exam table with your feet in stirrups, and a doctor is inserting instruments into your uterus, you will be glad you took the time to check around beforehand. But if you don't have the luxury of making a choice, at least you will be armed with enough information to ask the questions that will help you avoid unsafe—or even life-threatening—situations.

CHAPTER FOUR

Back to the Bad Old Days?

BECAUSE OF significant advances in abortion technology and the widespread availability of legal abortion, many people have forgotten what life was like when abortion was illegal. Dr. Jerry Hulka, Professor of Obstetrics and Gynecology at the University of North Carolina School of Medicine, describes what he saw on an ongoing basis as an intern, a resident, and then as an attending physician, in hospitals in Pittsburgh from 1957 to 1967. "In one hospital, we had a special ward that was always filled with women who had infections and perforations from illegal abortions," he says. Dr. Hulka often assisted Dr. Sam Barr, a senior physician on the staff, with these cases. **Dr. Barr ultimately wrote a book[1] about the need for abortion reform, in which he recalled one unforgettable case:**

> I'll never forget one patient; she was 32 years old and the mother of two children. She was admitted through the emergency room [and] wouldn't say anything except that she thought she ought to get help as soon as possible...Her symptoms were relatively mild. Her pelvis was moderately tender and her uterus was only slightly enlarged, but she did have a positive pregnancy test. There was one other finding: a small puncture point with a little bit of bleeding at the entrance of her uterus....I suspected that either she had tried to abort herself, or someone else had done it to her. When I checked on her a little later, I had to press the

97

point of asking her what had happened because she had visibly weakened.

"I had to do it," she said. "I went to this lady who put a coat hanger up in me. She told me not to panic, but if there was some real problem, don't say anything but go to the emergency room. I figured that blood coming out whenever I went to the bathroom was a problem and I got real scared."

With luck, I thought, the worst diagnosis would be that this woman's bladder had been perforated. That would not be pleasant, but hopefully there wasn't any major systemic problem. I started massive antibiotic treatment immediately, beginning with several transfusions to replace the blood she had lost...[but] three hours later I learned I was wrong....First, the laboratory reported that preliminary studies indicated an infection with gas gangrene. Then, the nurse on the floor said that the patient looked just awful—she wasn't bleeding much but she had a lot of difficulty breathing. I ran to the floor and found her slipping rapidly into heart failure. The professor who headed our program came in to assist, but everything that 20 skilled people could contribute did not help. The gangrene bacteria were destroying her red blood cells. That vital fluid was turning into little more than red water.* Her heart couldn't handle it and her body was dying....The last thing I remember her saying to me was, "I know you tried. Figure some way to tell my kids. They won't understand at all. Tell them for me somehow. I don't want them to think me bad." She lost consciousness and then, a little bit later, just before dawn, she died.

---

* Today, this problem would probably be recognized as *disseminated intravascular coagulation (DIC)*, in which the blood loses its ability to clot. See pages 233-234 for more information on this rare but serious complication.

Dr. Hulka was one of the doctors who tried to help this woman. He vividly remembers her pain and her death, and says that similar cases occurred on a daily basis because of repressive abortion laws. "Women and doctors have forgotten about these deaths," he says. "Unless something is done quickly to stem the tide of regressive legislation, we are going to start seeing such unnecessary deaths again."

The nameless woman in the above story left two children, perhaps quite young ones, who had to face life without the love and protection of their mother. We will never know how her children fared in life, but we do know that losing a mother is perhaps the most devastating psychological event children can face, and putting them at a severe disadvantage growing up.

Holly, who is now in her early seventies, and raised three children of her own, lost her mother to a self-induced abortion in 1922.

When my older sister was seven, I was five, and my baby sister was two, we lived with our parents in one big room in Pittsburgh. When our mother, who was 28 years old at the time, got pregnant for the fourth time, there simply wasn't room for another child, so our dad went to the drugstore and got some medicine. I don't know what it was, but she took it. Later, she started hemorrhaging so he took her to the hospital. She lived for a few days, but one night, Dad came home and was crying and said that our mother was dead. I remember seeing her laid out in the living room of my aunt's house. We just couldn't understand why it had happened. In the months after her death, our father drank heavily and had a hard time holding down a job. There was no money, so he sent us to an orphanage. The building was on the top of a high hill, and every day for seven

*years, my sisters and I looked down the hill,
waiting for Dad to come visit us. He came, but only
about every six months.*

During the 1960s, Dr. Alex Brickler, an African-American gynecologist in Tallahassee, Florida, took care of numerous young women at the student health service at Florida A&M University, which was at the time Florida's only public university for African-American students. **Dr. Brickler remembers how difficult those times were for doctors in smaller communities, yet how common abortion was.**

> *It was an open secret who did abortions in town.
> There was even a doctor who had his own hos-
> pital where he did abortions, but the laws were
> very threatening, and we were at risk if we even
> referred patients to him. In any event, the results
> weren't necessarily good. At the time, the favored
> method of abortion was inserting a catheter, a thin
> rubber tube, into the uterus to precipitate a miscar-
> riage. That was almost a formal invitation to an
> infection, and I treated many. I particularly
> remember several young undergraduates who
> came in with massive infections. These young
> women, 18 or 19 years old, were poised on the
> threshold of life. They had everything ahead of
> them—their lives, their careers, their families, but
> we simply couldn't save them.*

In the days before abortion was legal, many doctors undertook enormous personal and professional risks to do abortions. Dr. Ruth Barnett, a Portland, Oregon, naturopath, was one of them. Barnett learned to do abortions while she was secretary for a female gynecologist in Portland, and later, as a receptionist for Dr. George Watts, a prominent gynecologist who also did abortions in Portland. "Soon I was interviewing patients, preparing them for surgery, sterilizing the instruments and keeping them in order....After a time, [Dr. Watts] began instructing me in the painstaking details of his technique." Dr. Watts encouraged Barnett to go to chiropractic school in order to become licensed, which she did, and later he lent her money to buy a rival practice down the hall from his own office.

Dr. Watts moved to Los Angeles and became a partner in an ambitious chain of clinics that not only did abortions but trained other doctors to do them as well. The chain spread all over the West Coast, but since the profits were technically illegal, eventually its partners ran afoul of the Internal Revenue Service. All of the clinics were busted, and Barnett, now Dr. Barnett, watched in horror as her benefactor, and other doctors and nurses he worked with, were tried and sent to San Quentin Penitentiary.

Dr. Barnett herself was arrested four times during the 1950s and 1960s, and was finally convicted and sent to prison when she was 70 years old and ill with cancer. In her autobiography, *They Weep On My Doorstep*,[2] Dr. Barnett, reviews her gutsy, unconventional career and provides a revealing glimpse into the lives of underground abortionists and the plight of the women they served. **After her second arrest in the early 1950s, she stood in her clinic, which was about to be closed, and reminisced about one particular patient.**

> *She was only 15, slightly built, blue-eyed, blond and innocent, with immature breasts poking small rounded points into her sweater. She seemed numb as I questioned her. She said she had been raped.*
>
> *"Who raped you?" I asked.*
> *"My father. He was drunk."*

"When?"

"Maybe seven months ago."

Examination corroborated her statement. She had been pregnant too long. When I said that an abortion would be impossible, she asked, almost tonelessly, "What can I do?"

"Nothing," I said. "You'll have to have the child."

"My own father's baby?"

I could only nod. My throat was too choked for speech. She arose, went to the door, stood there a moment, turned toward me as though she were going to say something further. But she said nothing. She was weeping. She shook her head once and left. The next morning the police fished her body from the Willamette River.

Dr. Barnett's career spanned almost 50 years, from 1918 until her final conviction and imprisonment in 1966. During that time she performed more than 40,000 abortions, not only for the women of Portland and its environs, but for women from San Francisco, Seattle, Boise, Salt Lake City, and other West Coast towns. In addition, she notes, "A great many cases came from a prominent Catholic gynecologist who would tell women who insisted on an abortion to 'go to the Broadway Building and ask for Dr. Ruth.' "

Death wasn't the only consequence of poorly done illegal abortions. **Uterine infections frequently resulted in lifelong pain or infertility, as it did for Janice, a Boston schoolteacher, whose life was dramatically changed one night on her kitchen table.**

In the early 1950s, we already had three children, and I was planning to go back to teaching so we could build an addition to our home. When I found out I was pregnant, my husband and I were both very upset because, if I didn't go back to work we wouldn't have the money for the construction. I didn't know what to do, but a friend of my husband's said that he knew someone who could "take care of things." I had heard stories about "kitchen table" abortions and initially refused, but after a week of arguments, I agreed to have an abortion. On Friday night, after the children had been put to bed, a woman who my husband's friend said was a nurse came to the house. I drank a lot of sherry beforehand and don't remember much about the abortion, except that it did indeed take place on the kitchen table. During the night I began having severe pelvic pains, but was too embarrassed to call my own gynecologist. He was very thorough and also very conservative, and I thought he might ask too many questions, so I went to a doctor recommended by a friend. He said that I must have had a "puncture," and would have to have a hysterectomy. During the surgery, he also removed part of my bowel, saying later that it had been damaged as well. My recovery from the surgery took a long time, and afterward I developed chronic pelvic pain. I complained so much that my doctor finally did an exploratory operation and found that I had "adhesions," [a sort of fibrous, internal scar tissue] around my bowel as a result of the first surgery. A second surgery removed part of my small intestine, leaving me with chronic digestive difficulties and a very limited diet. Up until the night of my abortion I was a healthy person. Afterward, I became a medical case—always in pain, always in the hospital for something.

Janice's case never made headlines, yet her life was profoundly changed, both by her abortion and by her hysterectomy, which may or may not have been necessary by today's medical standards. But she was lucky. She got medical help, and did not bleed to death, as many women did, in their bathrooms, in shabby hotel rooms, or in hospitals, where even the best of medical help often came too late.

THE ABORTION HANDBOOK

The U.S. abortion reform movement was fueled by the work of a number of highly visible activists who published pamphlets, organized demonstrations, established abortion referral services, taught classes on abortion, and worked through the courts to normalize and legalize abortion. The work of these activists was supported by a legion of unsung heroes: doctors who risked their licenses to provide women with safe procedures; therapists, social workers, and clergy who risked their livelihoods making reliable referrals; and the friends, family members, and occasionally strangers who supported women through days of pain, fear, and uncertainty that all too often followed surreptitious abortions. (See Suggested Reading on page 259 for more information on the compelling history of the abortion reform movement.)

But waiting for the courts to respond was like waiting for Samuel Beckett's eternally truant Godot. He was always anticipated, but no one seemed to know the precise hour of his arrival. So, while activists pressed ahead on various fronts in the late 1960s, a few women working at the grassroots level decided to take things into their own hands. Lana Clarke Phelan, a Long Beach, California, housewife, Pat Maginnis, a medical technician from San Francisco, and Rowena Gurner, a Bay Area activist, who became known as "the Army of Three," were among the most resolute of these activists.

"We were working all the time, traveling and lecturing," Lana remembers. "But it was like pushing on fog. Just when you thought you had made some progress, things just collapsed before your eyes." Pat and Rowena taught classes about abortion in the San Francisco Bay area, and openly courted arrests. To their dismay, they found that the police were reluctant to make arrests, because they didn't want to provide opportunities to challenge existing laws. Feeling very frustrated, Pat began writing down information from the classes on self-abortion and showed it to Lana.

"I thought it was too technical," says Lana. "It assumed a lot of information on the part of the reader. I thought it should be more practical." Lana took over the book, hammering it out on her portable typewriter every night. "I tried to keep it light, while tears were running down my face," Lana says. "I was so angry at all the authority men had, and they were not using it in our best interests." She finished a draft in six weeks and took it to two gynecologists who said, *"Get that book in print!"*

Lana quickly found a publisher who "came to the house with a contract and didn't leave any of his money behind when he left with the contract signed." But money didn't matter to Lana as much as getting the book in print. And *The Abortion Handbook*[3], published in 1969, quickly became an underground classic. Lana estimates that it went through five printings, selling over 50,000 copies. "Once I even saw copies of it on a newsstand in Penn Station in New York City, so I knew it had gotten around," she remarks.

The Abortion Handbook is surely one of the most creative, irreverent, and subversive documents of American feminism. In a voice that is at the same time empathetic, militant, and provocative, it counsels women to give their doctors "a large piece of your mind for his gross neglect of your health, and his sworn medical duty, in forcing you into underground or self-abortion paths." *The Abortion Handbook* speaks directly to women, exhorting them to take control of their lives before they lose them. Sadly, the bulk of the information it contains is all too relevant today.

"THIS IS JANE FROM WOMEN'S LIBERATION"

One of the most widely known examples of women taking things into their own hands was Jane, the now legendary group of women that took over an abortion referral service in Chicago, turned it into a booming abortion business, and ultimately, learned to do the abortions themselves.

From 1964 until 1968, Heather Booth, one of the founders of the Chicago women's liberation movement, and some of her friends, ran an ad hoc abortion referral service out of Heather's dormitory room at the University of Chicago. One day, Heather called some women together, talked about the politics of abortion, trained them to counsel, handed over her contact sheets, and left. "I was ready to move on," she says.

"That was the real beginning of Jane," says a woman we'll call Leslie, a long-time member of the group. Right away, the women in the group decided that the system they had inherited needed improvement.

"We got the calls, then turned the women's names over to abortionists, and didn't have any contact again until after the procedure. They came back alive. That's about all we knew," Leslie recalls. "They waited on street corners to be picked up then were blindfolded. It must have been so scary. From the beginning, we tried to make the experience different. We explained what it was going to be like, how it was going to feel, what the basic m.o. was."

Leslie remembers receiving counseling calls at her home. "When you said, 'This is Jane from Women's Liberation,' you could hear an audible sigh of relief."

The first thing that needed improvement was the price: The abortions were expensive—from $600 to $1,000—and that was out of the reach of many poor women. So the group decided to attempt to gain some control over the price by cutting a deal with one of their doctors. The deal worked. In return for volume, he lowered the price to about $500. Then, in late 1970, at the end of the second year of the Service (as Jane was also called), the group found out that the man, like many others who did illegal abortions, was not a doctor. The revelation created an enormous philosophical crisis among the group. Some women felt betrayed. Others left. Others felt liberated.

"That was when we realized that if he could do abortions and wasn't a doctor, then we could learn to do them ourselves," Leslie says. Still, nothing happened for a while. Finally, one of the women in the group pressured the abortionist to share his skills.

"He was reluctant at first," Leslie recalls, "but then he agreed. A few other women learned from him, and by the fall of 1971, we were doing all of the abortions ourselves. Mostly we learned in stages, first by assisting—up to and including dilation—and then doing more, as each of us became more comfortable with the procedure.

"Doing the abortions ourselves had enormous advantages," Leslie continues. "We dropped the price to $100 or whatever the woman could pay. The average was about $40." By this time the group was doing 20 to 30 abortions a day, three days a week, and continued to use the standard D&C procedure they had learned from their abortionist for women who were up to 14 weeks from their last menstrual periods.

"We always had to be on our toes. Anything could happen—and it did," Leslie confesses. "Often we improvised. For example, hemorrhages could often be dealt with on the spot by applying ice or giving ergotrate (a drug used to help the uterus contract)." When emergencies occurred, they drove the woman to the hospital emergency ward.

"We took women to the door, but it was too dangerous to the group for anyone to go in with them, so we just helped them get their stories straight and told them to call us when they got home. 'Act dumb,' we told them. 'That's what doctors expect from women.'"

Jane had a policy of never turning away any woman who wanted to terminate her pregnancy, as long as the counselors felt that she wouldn't be too upset by the procedure. But like doctors of that era, they didn't have the technology to do late second trimester abortions.

"If women were too far along, we just induced a miscarriage by breaking the waters," Leslie recalls. Afterward, women whose miscarriages had been induced went home and waited, an ordeal which, Leslie notes, "often took incredible bravery." She remembers one teenager who called in every half hour while her father slept in the next room, asking in a whisper, "What do I do now?"

Considering the volume of business that passed through the Service, it is astonishing that the bust didn't come sooner.

"In the early days, a number of our clients were policemen's wives, girlfriends, or daughters," Leslie says. "After a while, we began to feel sort of protected." One treasured anecdote about the hands-off attitude of the police describes an incident that took place in the predominantly white Lincoln Park neighborhood:"The entrance to the building where the abortions were being done was on a side street, and a young African-American woman was walking up and down the street, looking in vain for the address. She was surprised when a police car pulled up beside her, and the policeman pointed out the entrance on a side street nearby."

The bust occurred in May 1972. A relative of a woman who was scheduled for an abortion didn't feel comfortable with the arrangements and called the police.

"Two homicide detectives came in looking for 'the money and the man,'" Leslie remembers. "'He just jumped out the window,' somebody said. That was a great joke, since we were in a high rise."

In all, seven women were arrested. Some members dropped out in fear, but two weeks later, Jane was back in business. In the meantime, the group got women appointments at clinics they knew of in New York and Washington.

"We called in all the feminist chips in town and collected plane fare for those who couldn't afford it," Leslie says. "Women were going to get their abortions no matter what."

Jane operated until April of 1973, three months after the *Roe v. Wade* decision, by which time several legal clinics had opened in Chicago. Afterward, some of the group stayed together and with other women founded the Emma Goldman Women's Health Center, named after the famous anarchist who was one of the earliest advocates of birth control in the United States. The Emma Goldman operated until the mid-1980s on the north side of Chicago. [Laura Kaplan, a long-time member of the Service, is writing a history of Jane to be published by Pantheon in 1993.]

BACK TO THE FUTURE?

The stories in this chapter serve as a grim reminder of what life was like for many women and their families when abortion was illegal, and what it may be like again if repressive laws make abortion inaccessible once more.

The New Y

NEW YORK, TU

VOL. CXXII . No. 42,003

© 1973 The New York Times Company

LYNDON JOHNSON, 367
WAS ARCHITECT OF 'G

High Court Rules Aborti

The New

VOL. CXXXVIII ... No. 47,921   Copyright © 1989 The New York Times

NEW YO

SUPREME COURT, 5-4,
UPHOLDS SHARP S

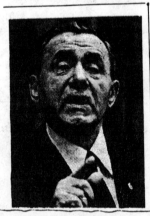

THE MAJORIT

RELIGIOUS DISPLAYS

In Menorah and Crèche Rulings, Court Takes Case-by-Case Tack

By LINDA GREENHOUSE
Special to The New York Times

WASHINGTON, July 3 — Drawing ever finer distinctions between permissible and impermissible Government commemorations of religion, the Su-

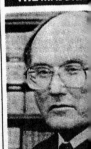

**Chief Justice
William H. Rehnqu**

"Nothing in the Con

rk **Times**

Weather: Partly sunny, mild ...
fair tonight. Sunny, mild tomorrow.
Temp. range: today 45-59; Monday
35-54. Full U.S. report on Page 76.

15 CENTS

UARY 23, 1973

'RESIDENT, IS DEAD;
AT SOCIETY' PROGRAM

Legal the First 3 Months

STRICKEN AT HOME

TION IS SHOCKED

ork **Times**

Late Edition

New York: Today: Limited hazy sun.
High 87. Tonight, evening showers possible. Low 70. Tomorrow, cloudy skies,
chance of a shower. High 86. Yesterday:
High 86, low 69. Details are on page 58.

SDAY, JULY 4, 1989   50 cents beyond 75 miles from New York City, except on Long Island.   35 CENTS

RROWING ROE V. WADE,
'E LIMITS ON ABORTIONS

THE DISSENT

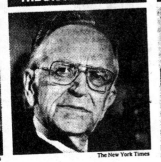

The New York Times

Justice Harry A. Blackmun

"I fear for the future. I fear for the
liberty and equality of the millions

THE MISSOURI LAW

These are the restrictions on
abortion in the Missouri law
that was upheld by the Supreme Court yesterday:

Public Hospital Ban

Public hospitals or other
taxpayer-supported facilities may not be used for performing abortions not necessary to save life, even if no
public funds are spent.

Public Employee Ban

Public employees, including
doctors, nurses and other

CHANGE IN COURSE

A Right Is Challenged —
Justices Accept More
Cases on the Issue

By LINDA GREENHOUSE
Special to The New York Times

WASHINGTON, July 3 — The Supreme Court today gave states the
right to impose sharp new restrictions
on abortion in a splintered decision indicating that a majority of the Court no
longer considers abortion to be a funda-
mental constitutional right.

A NOTE TO THE READER

All home health-care procedures, including menstrual extraction, can, under some circumstances, carry certain risks, even if performed correctly. The information in this book is intended to be for the elucidation of the reader, **but does not constitute an adequate set of instructions**. Indeed, the central message of the chapters on menstrual extraction is that women without specialized medical backgrounds can learn to perform it. but their training *must* involve working with a group over a period of time, learning directly about women's reproductive anatomy and function; it *must* include self-education, utilizing medical texts and journals; it *must* include independent research into abortion availability in the immediate area and beyond; it *must* include locating medical personnel to provide consultation and assistance; it *must* involve a group of women who are committed to in-depth discussion of the struggle for women's reproductive rights and periodic reassessment of the group's goals; and it *must* include, if at all possible, personal observation of clinical abortion, to become adequately acquainted with the differences and similarities between menstrual extraction and clinical procedures.

Benefit-risk assessments will vary, situation by situation. The authors have attempted to explain which risks, although statistically low, might possibly be encountered by a group or an individual, and which other risks are quite rare, but can be very serious when they do occur. The reader must then evaluate the risks and the benefits, depending on the situation in which she finds herself, in order to make an informed decision.

CHAPTER FIVE

The Development of Menstrual Extraction

MENSTRUAL EXTRACTION (ME) was developed as a technique to help women maintain control over their menstrual cycles, and hence, over their reproductive lives. On or about the day that a woman expects her menstrual period, the contents of the uterus are gently suctioned out, lightening and greatly shortening the expected period. If an egg has been fertilized within the preceding weeks, it will be suctioned out as well. Dealing as it does with normal bodily functions, ME is not a medical treatment—but a home health-care technique, similar in many ways to self-catheterization, at-home bladder instillations, and other health-maintenance routines.

The tabloids and the electronic media have labeled menstrual extraction "self-abortion" or "do-it-yourself abortion," but these terms are misleading. First of all, due to the location of the uterus, it is virtually impossible for a woman to do ME on herself. To do the procedure safely and correctly, a woman needs the help of one or more women who are trained and experienced in ME. In this sense, it is no more appropriate to label ME "self-abortion" than it is to call home birth "self-birth." Lorraine Rothman, one of the developers of ME, explains that the name *menstrual extraction* was chosen "because it is a very literal description of the process."

THE DEVELOPMENT OF
MENSTRUAL EXTRACTION

In 1970, Carol Downer, a housewife and mother of six young children, was working on the abortion committee of the Los Angeles chapter of the National Organization for Women (NOW). "One woman in the group was working in an illegal abortion clinic in Santa Monica," Carol recalls. "She had figured out that abortion wasn't as difficult as it was made out to be, and suggested that we do abortions ourselves."

One day Carol went to the clinic with that woman and the woman's daughter, who was going to have an IUD inserted. Suddenly Carol found herself in the procedure room, where the younger woman was already on the examination table with a speculum in place.

"I got a glimpse of her cervix and was completely bowled over," Carol remembers. "It was such a shock to see how simple and accessible our anatomy is. At that moment, everything clicked for me. I had read *The Abortion Handbook*, and realized that if women just had some basic information about their bodies, they could take care of themselves and wouldn't have to depend on back alley abortionists."

Carol and a small group of activists organized an event billed as a "Self-Help Clinic" at Everywoman's Bookstore in Venice Beach on April 7, 1971. "To us, 'self-help' meant taking control of our bodies and our health care," she says.

Lorraine Rothman, a public school teacher in Orange County, just south of Los Angeles, and herself the mother of four, recalls the first Self-Help Clinic meeting vividly. "I had read an article in Everywoman's Newspaper that made it sound like women in L.A. were doing abortions. I thought, 'Of course. What did women do before they had doctors? It can't be that hard. Let's just stop the frustration and humiliation of trying to persuade the powers that be to legalize abortion. Let's just take back the technology, the tools, the skills, and whatever else we need.'"

In the weeks before the first Self-Help Clinic, Carol and a few other women from the group had visited an underground abortion clinic run by Harvey Karman in Santa Monica. Karman, who the group later found out was not a medical doctor, was one of the most active proponents of a new, non-traumatic suction abortion technique that made use of a flexible plastic cannula (a thin tube about the size of a soda straw that can be inserted into the uterus) and a hand-held syringe used to create suction and to collect the uterine contents. Proponents of this technique generally eschewed the use of a curette, a razor-sharp, spoon-like instrument used for D&Cs (see illustration on page 82).

At the first Self-Help Clinic meeting, about 30 women sat in a circle on the floor. When Carol's turn came to speak, she said she had something special she wanted to share with the group. She climbed up on a desk, inserted a plastic speculum into her vagina, and demonstrated to the amazed onlookers how accessible a woman's cervix (the neck of the uterus that protrudes into the vagina) was. "After that, the discussion took a different turn," Lorraine remembers. "We talked about taking charge of our own health care."

One woman had brought a cannula and a large plastic syringe (minus the needle) from Karman's abortion clinic and showed it to the group. Lorraine immediately felt that the device had two obvious weaknesses. "For one thing, there was no mechanism to prevent air from being accidentally pumped back into the uterus—which was one of the big scary things about illegal abortion," she says. "For another, the uterine contents passed directly through the cannula into the syringe. If the syringe got full, the cannula would have to be removed, so that the syringe could be emptied. This was clumsy to handle and caused additional discomfort for the woman. I thought there must be a better way."

Lorraine took the apparatus home and spent the next week haunting hardware stores, grocery stores, chemistry labs and aquarium shops. She brought her version of the device to the next Self-Help Clinic meeting. This modified device consisted of a cannula and a large (50 or 60cc) syringe for pumping suction, but Lorraine's version had two tubes, one leading from the cannula into a collection jar, and the other leading from the syringe into the jar. When pumped, the syringe created a vacuum inside the jar, and the contents of the uterus were sucked into the jar, instead of into the syringe. An automatic two-way bypass valve, which Lorraine located in a scientific mail-order catalog, prevents air from being pumped back into the uterus.* She dubbed the device "Del-Em."

"We were on that device like ducks on a June bug," Carol remembers. "Word about this new technique got around very quickly. We were learning to estimate the size of a pregnant and non-pregnant uterus, and got a lot of practice. But for women who were in fact pregnant, we were getting too many incomplete abortions and we wanted to know more."

Carol had heard about Dr. Franz Koomey, the doctor in Washington state who had led the fight to legalize abortion there and who used paramedics in his clinics. "I mentioned Koomey to Lorraine one evening, and she just said, *'Let's go!'*" Without so much as doing the laundry, the two took off the next morning in the Rothman family

---

* If air is accidentally pumped into the uterus, it will probably pass through the egg tubes into the abdominal cavity, causing gas-like discomfort or pain. If any air accidentally enters the blood stream, this can result in a fatal air embolism.

station wagon for the Pacific Northwest. "I just told my husband that I would need the car for a couple of weeks. I was afraid if I *asked* he might say no," Lorraine remembers with a laugh.

Carol and Lorraine worked in Koomey's clinic for several days observing abortions. "Dr. Koomey had a well-deserved reputation as an activist, but we were shocked that he still used curettes and large, stiff cannulas which required that the cervix be dilated a lot before they could be inserted," Carol says. "Women were given no anesthetic, and, consequently, had a lot of pain." (Unanesthetized procedures were a prominent hallmark of illegal abortions, because women were usually required to leave the premises quickly, and to do so, they had to be mobile.)

One day, Koomey invited Carol and Lorraine to do procedures under his supervision. They found the D&C procedure without anesthetic excessively brutal. "At the end of the day, we had a lot of experience, but we were more convinced than ever that the suction procedure was the way to go," Lorraine says.

Menstrual extraction made its public debut at the National Organization for Women conference in Santa Monica in August, 1971. The conference organizers thought that the concept was too shocking and refused to grant the group exhibit space. Undeterred, the West Coast Sisters, as they were now known, put up leaflets announcing demonstrations of the procedure in their hotel room.

"Women flocked in!" Lorraine reports. "The first day we packed in twenty or more at a time for demonstrations. The next day they were lined up in the hallway. We did demonstrations all day until we were exhausted." Women left the ME marathon with plastic speculums in little brown bags, and the Self-Help group acquired a national mailing list. From the list, Carol and Lorraine, put together a national tour. Traveling by bus and selling speculums transported in boxes marked "toys," they hit 23 cities in six weeks, spreading the word about self-examination, menstrual extraction and self-empowerment.

Lolly Hirsch, a housewife and mother of five from Stamford, Connecticut, was one of the women who attended a menstrual extraction demonstration at the Santa Monica NOW conference. Lolly and her daughter Jeanne immediately saw the implications of menstrual extraction. "The self-empowerment aspects were just so phenomenal," Jeanne observes. "My mother and I, and later, my sisters, were definitely committed." In the next 10 years, Lolly and Jeanne started a number of self-help groups in the Stamford area, got on the college lecture circuit, and began publishing a newsletter, wryly entitled "The Monthly Extract: An Irregular Periodical."

"Ultimately, several women we met on the tour migrated to Los Angeles, and joined the struggle," Carol Downer recalls. "They all shared our vision of wanting to change women's lives, and they had the will and the wits to do it." The group, which had lost some original members and gained some new ones, founded the Women's Abortion Referral Service with the highly appropriate acronym of WARS. They made an arrangement with a doctor who worked at a hospital where a staff psychiatrist rubber-stamped "applications" WARS brought in and the abortions were done quite openly.

Then, suddenly, on January 22, 1973, after more than two years of internal rancor, indecision, and equivocation, the United States Supreme Court announced its decision in the case of *Roe v. Wade*.

"That abruptly changed everything," Carol says. "We borrowed some money, hired a doctor, and opened a clinic." In March of 1973, WARS became the Women's Choice Clinic of the Los Angeles Feminist Women's Health Center. In July, Lorraine opened a sister clinic in Santa Ana, near her home in Orange County. Other Feminist

Women's Health Centers opened in the next two or three years in Chico and San Diego, California, Portland, Oregon, Tallahassee, Florida, and Atlanta, and later, Yakima, Washington, ultimately forming the Federation of Feminist Women's Health Centers.

For the time being, which right then seemed like forever, Carol, Lorraine, and their cohorts focused their attention on managing legal abortion clinics and working on a broad range of reproductive health concerns—safe second trimester abortions, woman-centered childbirth, the cervical cap, and many others—at the local, state, and national levels. Menstrual extraction went on the back burner. Women still learned the technique and a small number of them, perhaps as many as a thousand at any one time, maintained their skills, "just in case."

After *Roe v. Wade* legalized abortion, providers sprung up nationwide, and by the mid-1970s, about 75% of U.S. counties had an identifiable abortion provider. Because of the widespread availability of abortion, doctors assumed that there was no longer any need for women to be concerned about taking care of themselves, and were sometimes critical of the continuing interest in menstrual extraction, especially since there were no studies on its safety and effectiveness.

To counter this criticism, Carol and Lorraine contacted various research organizations in search of funding for a study. The one expression of interest came from Dr. Christopher Tietze, the preeminent expert on abortion and contraception at the Population Council, a social policy organization funded by the Rockefeller family.

"Dr. Tietze was quite intrigued by ME and our experience with it, and encouraged us to submit a proposal," Carol recalls. "We did submit one, but the Foundation declined to fund it on the grounds that it did not fund 'direct services.'" Menstrual extraction became a practice maintained by a small cadre of women who worked tirelessly for legal abortion, but who continued to believe in the enduring importance of self-empowerment.

WHEN BIRTH CONTROL FAILS

In early 1977, when the Allende regime was overthrown in Chile, a group of prominent women's health activists, which included feminist author Barbara Ehrenreich, Sally Guttmacher, a well-known women's health advocate and professor of Health Education at New York University, and the late Bobbye Ortiz, a long-time Associate Editor of *The Monthly Review*, formed Action for Women in Chile (WIC) out of concern for the conditions in prisons for women political prisoners. This group began working with a Chilean group that had asked for information on abortion. The Chilean women were particularly interested in finding self-help techniques that might be useful for women political prisoners who were raped in prison. Ehrenreich passed their request on to Carol Downer and her co-workers. "We were aware of the drastic measures that women sometimes resort to in order to control their lives. We also knew that with sufficient information, women had safely and successfully aborted themselves," says Suzann Gage, a health worker in the Los Angeles clinic and illustrator of the Center's books on women's health care. "I was inspired to put that information in visual form so it could be understood by any woman, regardless of what language she spoke."

Suzann spoke with women who had done menstrual extraction, and with others who were familiar with herbs and other techniques of pregnancy termination. She also mined the pages of *The Abortion Handbook* (see page 104) for information on self-help techniques. After working all day in the clinic, Suzann stayed up nights drawing and writing explanatory text. When it was finished, the text with illustrations was staple-bound in an easily reproducible format and transmitted to the women at WIC, who then forwarded it to their contacts in Chile.

"This book was deliberately very bare bones," Suzann recalls. "It was intended only for women who were committed self-helpers. And yet at the same time, we wanted to preserve this information for women who had no other options open to them."

Over the years, and in various formats, this information has made its way to women throughout the world in Chile, Mexico, Nicaragua, most European countries, Australia, New Zealand, Japan and Iran. In 1979, the copy was typeset and published by Speculum Press as *When Birth Control Fails*. The book quickly became an underground classic, and enjoyed a brief revival after the *Webster* decision in 1989, but is now out of print.

OTHER USES FOR MENSTRUAL EXTRACTION

The early proponents of menstrual extraction gained valuable information about their own bodies and menstrual cycles, information that was otherwise only available, if it existed at all, in abstruse medical texts. They found that they could shorten and significantly diminish a normal heavy period, which could be a boon to female athletes, travelers, campers, executives, honeymooners—any woman to whom a long or heavy period might pose a substantial inconvenience. They also found that when employed on a regular basis, menstrual extraction could be used as birth control, similar to an IUD, to prevent the implantation of a fertilized egg about two weeks after fertilization. In short, they found that being able to safely extract the contents of the uterus provided a measure of reproductive control that few women had even dreamed of.

Val, a massage therapist, combined menstrual extraction with fertility awareness for several years.

Fertility awareness employs the observation of cervical secretions, basal body temperature, and a host of bodily signs to pinpoint ovulation. Knowing the precise time of ovulation can be useful in avoiding pregnancy, by abstaining from intercourse until about 24 hours after ovulation. Fertility awareness can also be useful in enhancing the chances of getting pregnant, by identifying the fertile time and coordinating it with intercourse or donor insemination.

My periods were always somewhat irregular, coming anywhere from 27 to 35 days. Fertility awareness gave me much more information about and control over my cycle than I ever dreamed possible, but there were still times when I just couldn't tell when I had ovulated. Because of the variability of my cycle, I spent a lot of time in suspense, wondering if my period was ever going to come. After I began doing menstrual extraction, if my period didn't come by day 35, I would called my self-help group and have an extraction. Once it turned out that I was pregnant, but the extraction still felt so normal—as normal as getting my period when I wanted it.

There have also been reports of instances when menstrual extraction provided a life-saving function. Margaret, who was among the first women to learn menstrual extraction, recalls one such situation.

It was 2:00 in the morning during a raging blizzard when I got a call from a midwife I knew. One of her clients had just had a late miscarriage and was bleeding heavily. The midwife had arrived in a jeep several hours earlier, but now couldn't get out, and she was sure that an ambulance wouldn't make it up the long, icy hill. She also knew that if the woman didn't stop bleeding soon, she would probably need a transfusion. She thought that emptying the uterus mechanically would make it contract, and curtail the bleeding, so she called and asked if I would be willing to try a menstrual extraction. I got dressed and went, but halfway up the hill my car went off the road, so I walked the rest of the way. I did the extraction and moved the cannula quite vigorously, hoping that the stimulation would increase prostaglandin production enough to make the uterus contract. It worked! In about 45 minutes or so, the bleeding slowed to an acceptable level. The next day, when the road was cleared, the midwife took the woman to the hospital, where a doctor examined her and said she didn't need any further treatment.

Menstrual extraction clearly has a variety of uses, and consequently, has significant implications for women's health. The next section reveals how this simple technique has been adapted on a global scale to save the lives of many women who would otherwise be at the mercy of untrained technicians and dangerous folk methods of fertility control.

MENSTRUAL REGULATION IN THE DEVELOPING WORLD

At the same time that menstrual extraction was developing in California, international family planning activists began using a nearly identical method of fertility control in developing countries. The technique has had a variety of names: "minisuction," "menstrual induction," and "menstrual aspiration." However, the term most widely used today is menstrual regulation (MR). Like menstrual extraction, the procedure is often done without a laboratory test to confirm pregnancy. MR can also be used for teaching women about their anatomy and fertility, diagnosing uterine cancer, menstrual disorders, and infertility, and for completing self-induced or incomplete abortions.

One distinctive difference between the practices of menstrual regulation and menstrual extraction is in the equipment used. The Del-EM™ used in menstrual extraction is individually assembled, while the kit used in menstrual regulation is commercially produced and marketed.* With this kit, the uterine contents are suctioned directly through the cannula into a syringe, while with the Del-

*This device is manufactured by the International Projects Assistance Service (IPAS), P.O. Box 100, Carrboro, NC 27510, (800) 334-8446.

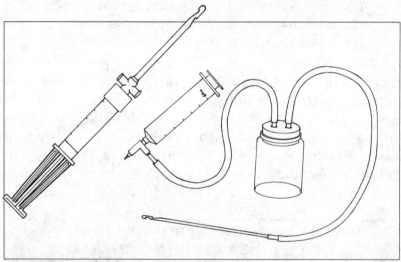

THE DEL-EM™ and a kit used for menstrual regulation in developing countries made by the International Projects Assistance Service (IPAS). The major difference is that the Del-Em™ collects the uterine contents in a jar, while it goes directly into the syringe of the IPAS kit. Both kits have a two-way bypass valve, to prevent air from entering the uterus.

Em™, the contents are suctioned through the cannula and a plastic tube about two feet long into a collection jar.

Early on, it became clear to medical professionals and family planning experts that paramedics and lay people with even minimal education could learn to use hand-generated suction devices safely and effectively. Today, training in most countries typically lasts from one to three weeks, occasionally longer, and is done on both a formal basis, including classroom lectures, demonstrations, and supervised practice; and on an informal basis, often consisting of demonstrations only. Trainees may observe from 10 to 20 procedures before beginning hands-on training, and then do up to 20 procedures under supervision before doing them on their own. Because of the lack of qualified trainers, and the demand for MR services, trainees sometimes begin doing unsupervised procedures without much hands-on instruction, but this is not recommended.[1]

In developing countries where health education and contraception are not widely available, women who fear they may be pregnant often seek to induce miscarriages with sticks, wires or other instruments, by drinking toxic substances, or by douching with harmful concoctions. In Nicaragua, for example, women commonly use wire from telephone cables to induce miscarriages. Others resort to poorly trained abortionists who often use stiff, unsterile instruments. As a result, at least 200,000 women die each year,[2] and many more are left infertile or with lifelong health problems. In addition, hundreds of thousands of children are left motherless or with a mother who may be too ill or disabled to provide for them adequately.

Many doctors who do menstrual regulation may use anesthesia, but in some clinics, the only anesthesia that is used is the comforting hand and soothing voice of a counselor. Zarina, a counselor at a women's clinic in Bangladesh, reports that most of the women who seek MR have already endured childbirth; most say the discomfort from the procedure is quite tolerable, even without anesthesia.

In practice, menstrual regulation is performed up to eight to 10 weeks from the last period, but in many countries, the procedure is also done up to 12 weeks from the last menstrual period. There are no reliable statistics on the rate of incomplete procedures in Bangladesh or other countries where MR is in use, but the rate of incompletes appears to be low, according to Zarina because "most women in these countries usually don't come in until they are eight to ten weeks from their last period, when it is easier to determine, by examining the tissue, whether or not an implantation has been missed."

Menstrual regulation is practiced throughout Latin America, Asia, in many African countries, and on a limited basis in the Middle East. *In every setting in which this technique has become accessible, the complication rate for self-*

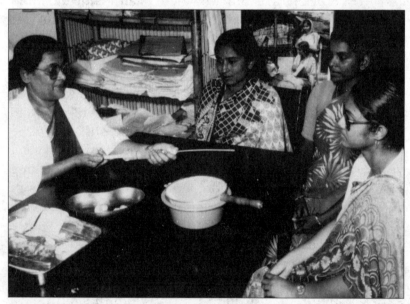

A COUNSELOR in a clinic in Bangladesh explaining the menstrual regulation procedure to three women. [Credit: John Paul Kay]

induced and poorly done abortions has been dramatically reduced. In Indonesia, for example, one study found that the rate of septic abortion was 80% higher in areas in which menstrual regulation (in this case, suction curettage) was not available, but that where MR was available, wards formerly reserved for cases of septic abortion were no longer necessary.[3] Clearly, if menstrual regulation were employed more widely, the health of many women—and the lives of many others—would be saved.

IN AN ERA that is hostile to reproductive freedom, menstrual extraction and other home health-care techniques (see Chapter 9) are profoundly relevant. Women may consciously choose to use menstrual extraction or to take herbs for fertility control for a variety of reasons. When used properly, these techniques are far safer than childbirth, and can put an end to the makeshift methods that desperate women have often used to prevent unwanted pregnancies.

CHAPTER SIX

Friendship Groups

IN THE LAST 20 years, perhaps 1,000 to 2,000 women in the United States have learned menstrual extraction by participating in small, close-knit groups based on friendship and a common goal of reclaiming control over their reproductive lives. These groups typically have from five to 10 members, and meet regularly—perhaps once a month or more often—to learn more about their bodies and their menstrual cycles, and to practice their skills. Groups that have been in existence for a long time may meet only occasionally, when one of the members chooses to have her period extracted.

THE SAFETY OF MENSTRUAL EXTRACTION

Trained practitioners—lay women, nurses, midwives, physicians assistants or other paramedics—have found menstrual extraction to be exceptionally safe. They maintain that because a smaller, more flexible cannula is used, because drugs are not routinely employed, and since conscientious practitioners have a commitment to be extremely careful and gentle, the risks of infection or perforation are exceedingly low.

Long-time practitioners have found that the safety of menstrual extraction is dependent upon three factors:

➡ practicing sterile technique, that is, knowing how to disinfect the cannula, the only instrument that enters the uterus, and accessory instruments.

➡ knowing the signs of a problem (discussed in detail on page 227).

➡ having a backup plan, i.e., having a formal or informal arrangement with a doctor or clinic, and knowing how to deal with paramedics and emergency room personnel in the unlikely event of a medical emergency.

We surveyed on-going self-help groups across the country, and interviewed representatives of three such groups, Gabriella, Emily, and Adrienne, asking them about their experiences and safety record. We also attended a self-help group meeting at the home of one group member.

TRAINING

Most self-help groups follow similar steps in learning menstrual extraction: reading as much as they can; discussing their feelings about menstrual extraction, abortion, and reproductive control; working out group policies and protocols; and assembling equipment and supplies. If possible, a group finds a mentor, a woman who is experienced with ME, to guide them through their first procedures and serve as an adviser as subsequent questions and problems arise. **Heather, who has been in a self-help group for about three years, shared her experiences in learning menstrual extraction with us.**

> We met about twice a month for three months before we actually did our first ME. At those meetings, we all did self-examination and uterine size checks. That alone was exhilarating, and we talked a lot about how we didn't want the entire focus to be on ME. We were very interested in herbal and barrier methods of birth control, particularly in the cervical cap, and some of the women who are lesbians were interested in donor insemi-

nation. A few of us had observed an ME before. Then, suddenly, two of us, Glenda and Rochelle, got pregnant. We didn't feel particularly ready, but we were in contact with Daphne, a woman who had been doing ME since the early 1970s, who was willing to step in and be our guide. At Glenda's extraction, Daphne did almost everything, explaining as she went, and only one of us tried moving the cannula a bit. It was a very easy ME. It took about 20 minutes, and Glenda had almost no discomfort. Rochelle's ME was harder because her uterus is very tilted. The procedure took several hours because Rochelle felt nauseous and threw up, so we took a lot of breaks. Daphne helped us through it, though, and we learned a lot. She said she thought it was good that we had had a difficult experience early, so we wouldn't think ME was always a piece of cake. After that, we did a lot of non-pregnant procedures and gradually gained confidence and skill.

Heather says that the next two and one-half years were a constant learning process. "We were taught to move the cannula and pump the syringe at the same time, but we found that we didn't really need to do them simultaneously. Doing them separately seems much more comfortable for the woman. We also discovered things like putting sterile lubricant on the tip of the cannula, which makes insertion go more smoothly."

In contrast to Heather's group, most new ME groups extract each other's periods for six months or more, acquiring skills and knowledge, before they attempt procedures when a woman is possibly pregnant.

Nicole echoes Heather's description of training as an on-going learning experience. She says that her group had to do a number of reaspirations until they learned a reliable method of judging if a procedure was complete. "One member of our group observed a few procedures done by an older group. They taught her to check for the placental sac at even three or four weeks of preganancy. That early, it's only about as big as the little toe-nail, but its's texture is very different from the chorionic villi." Nicole says that the sac is sturdy, but pliable, and is often attached to a clump of chorionic villi, but it doesn't tear easily like the chorionic villi does. The sac sometimes shreds, however, making it more difficult to identify. "Now that we look for the sac, as well as villi, we rarely have to reaspirate any more," she says.

A WOMAN'S REPRODUCTIVE ANATOMY

All of the women we spoke to agree that menstrual extraction cannot be done safely without a basic understanding of the location and function of a woman's reproductive anatomy—the ovaries, egg (Fallopian) tubes, uterus, and cervix.

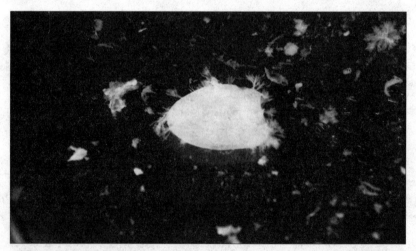

AT ABOUT SIX WEEKS of pregnancy, the sac, the membrane that eventually becomes the placenta, measures a little over an inch. This sac came out whole, and here is surrounded by the feathery chorionic villi.

Many women today still think of the uterus as remote and mysterious, but in fact it is not very far from the vaginal opening, and is actually quite accessible. The cervix, the neck of the uterus that protrudes into the

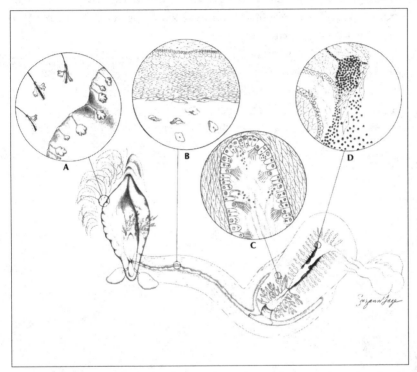

WHERE GENITAL SECRETIONS come from. In circle A, oil glands located on the inner lip of the clitoris (also called labia minora), secrete a light, milky fluid that is a key ingredient in the formation of the musky odor characteristic of the female genitals. In circle B, epithelial cells on the surface of the vaginal wall shed, and mix with vaginal secretions, causing them to be cloudy. In circle C, clear, viscous fertile mucous is manufactured in tiny glands located in the "crypts" of the cervical canal. Traces of fertile mucous appear four to five days before ovulation. The production increases and peaks a day or two before ovulation occurs. Most sperm die within two to three hours in normal vaginal acidity, but in the crypts of the cervical canal, nurtured by the alkaline fertile mucous, they can live for several days. When fertile mucous is present, you are at risk for getting pregnant. In circle D, blood pools in pockets called "venous lakes" near the surface of the uterine lining. When the pockets are full, they burst, mixing with epithelial cells from the lining of the uterus to form the menstrual flow.

vagina, can be seen by using a plastic speculum. When the speculum is inserted and locked in place, the cervix, looks like a little knob with a small hole or slit in the middle. This tiny hole, or *os* (Latin for opening), is where the menstrual blood and cervical mucus come out, and where the sperm go in. Some women's cervixes appear to be more flat and do not protrude very much.

The *os* leads to the cervical canal, a tunnel about an inch long, which in turn leads to the interior of the uterus. This canal, which is very narrow and tight, is lined with numerous dead-end passageways, often referred to as crypts, which house tiny glands that manufacture "fertile"

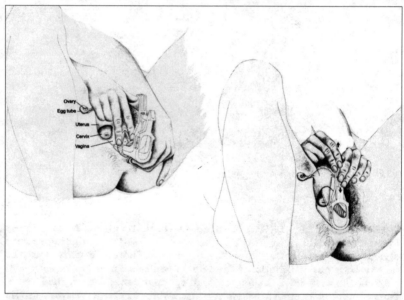

USING A PLASTIC SPECULUM. With one hand, spread the lips (labia) of the clitoris, and, holding the bills of the speculum together with the other, gently slide the closed bills into the vagina. Place one or two fingers of one hand on the short handle, and grasp the tall handle with two fingers and the thumb of the other hand. Now, with the two handles pressed tightly together, push down on the short handle and press up on the long one, until you hear one click. The speculum will actually open wider, but it is rarely necessary to use the other settings. The speculum will stay in place by itself, so that you have both hands free to use a light and mirror to look into the vagina.

mucus and "non-fertile" mucus. The alkaline fertile mucus, appears four to six days before ovulation and is produced in diminishing quantities for several days after ovulation has occurred. Once sperm have entered the cervical canal, and fertile mucus is present, they can remain alive and vigorous for three or four days, and thousands upon thousands of them continue their journey through the uterus into the egg tubes. This critical fact is why the Catholic "rhythm method" doesn't work.

The uterus itself is a tough, muscular organ shaped somewhat like a pear, and is about two and one-half to three inches long in its non-pregnant state. The uterine wall is densely lined with tiny, spiral-shaped arteries which become engorged with blood as ovulation approaches. Following ovulation, if no pregnancy occurs, the level of progesterone (the hormone that supports and nurtures a pregnancy) drops precipitously, and when the level has dipped far enough, the uterine arteries begin to constrict and burst, creating the menstrual flow.

If fertilization does occur, it happens within about 24 hours of ovulation, usually in the bottom third of the egg tube, and shortly the fertilized egg begins to divide. Within five to six days this clump of cells, now called a *blastocyst*, moves down into the uterus and within about a week begins producing its own progesterone, which helps it attach to the uterine wall.

The size of the uterus can be felt by another person doing a uterine size check (a two-handed or "bi-manual" exam). Two fingers of one hand in the vagina firmly press upward on the cervix, while three fingers of the other hand presses firmly on the abdomen just above the pubic hair line, so that the uterus is cupped between the two sets of fingers.

It takes a good deal of practice feeling different women's uteruses to become adept at judging whether a uterus is pregnant or not, and at estimating the number of weeks gestation of a pregnant uterus. (Even doctors who don't feel a lot of uteruses may not be very accurate at estimating gestational age.) Emily, a member of a different self-help group in the Midwest, says that being able to do accurate uterine size checks was one of the most difficult things for the women in her group to learn. "Thin women whose uteruses aren't tipped are the easiest to feel," she notes. "But you have to feel a lot of them in order to sort of 'memorize' the sizes at various stages of pregnancy." Emily

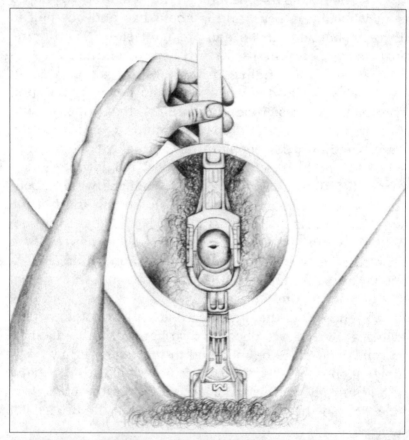

USING A FLASHLIGHT, goose-neck lamp, or other light source, a mirror, and a plastic speculum, you can easily see your cervix, the neck of the uterus that extends into the vagina. In this illustration, the *os*, the opening to the cervical canal, is clearly visible on the face of the cervix.

says that about half of the women in her group are les-
bians, and some of the heterosexual women don't have
regular sexual partners, so "we didn't get to feel a lot of
pregnant uteruses in the initial months of our training."

SPECULUMS

Plastic speculums cost less than a toothbrush (about $.60
each) and are standard equipment in many doctors'
offices. Like disposable syringes, douching equipment, and
enemas, they should be sold in all pharmacies.
Unfortunately, they are not widely available, so self-help
groups sometimes have difficulty finding a reliable source
of supply. Speculums come in small, medium, and long.
For use with menstrual extraction, the medium size might
appear to be the best, because it provides an optimal view
of the cervix, but given the 30 minutes or more it has to
remain in place, some women report being more comfortable using the small size.

Some groups buy speculums by the box at medical
supply houses, but others report getting smaller quantities
through hospitals, doctors' offices, medical labs, or
through friends who are nurses, medical students, technicians, or administrative workers. Emily points out that the
average self-help group probably doesn't need more than
25 to 30 speculums a year, and these can be disinfected
and reused indefinitely.

CANNULAS

Some self-help groups have found that the cannulas produced today are not as sturdy as they used to be, and recommend checking them before each use for cracks or
uneven edges. Policies differ on re-use. Groups that have a
reliable source of supply generally do not re-use cannulas,
but may store them in a safe place in case there is any dis-

ruption in availability. Groups whose supply is not so reliable say they may reuse cannulas up to five or six times, but check them carefully before each use. Emily, who worked in an abortion clinic for many years, reports that she has seen one or two instances where the tip of the cannula broke off inside the uterus and had to be removed with forceps. "That's why we check cannula tips—even the new ones—before use. And I don't mean just eyeball them. We bend them to look for obvious cracks."

DOING AN EXAM

"If a woman is fairly new to our group, before she has her first extraction, we review her health history and current health status," says Adrienne, a member of a group in

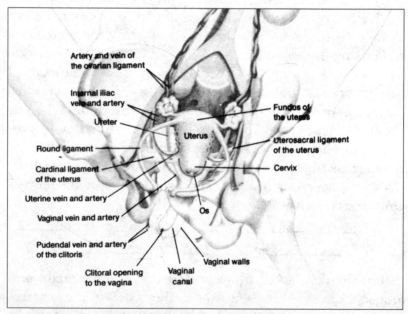

THE UTERUS IS ANCHORED in the pelvis by pairs of ligaments: the round ligaments, cardinal ligaments, and the uterosacral ligaments. The egg (Fallopian) tubes are attached to the top of the uterus, also called the fundus, and they curl around the ovaries. In this illustration the bladder, which is in front of the uterus, has been left out for a better view.

Northern California. "This can reveal any potential factors that might make the extraction difficult or risky. We're looking for conditions such as asthma, a history of pelvic inflammatory disease (PID), known allergic reactions, active I.V. drug use, epilepsy, or heart problems, that might be triggered by the stress sometimes caused by an extraction. If there is a potential problem that *anyone in the group feels uncomfortable with,* then we look at other alternatives for the woman and decide how to proceed. If she really wants to have her period extracted, we might consider taking extra precautions to avoid triggering an underlying health problem, or perhaps have her get further information from her doctor about the potential impact an extraction might have on a specific condition.

"If the health review does not reveal any contraindications to the procedure," Adrienne continues, "then several of us will do a uterine size check to ascertain if the uterus is its normal size, or if it is soft and enlarged, which would suggest that she might be pregnant. We would also ask her about any signs of pregnancy that she has noticed, and do a speculum exam to note the color of her cervix."

Making a determination of pregnancy can be more or less difficult depending on whether a woman has any changes in how she feels, or experiences changes in her body, and whether or not she menstruates regularly. See "Diagnosing Pregnancy" and "Birth Control Pills May Cloud the Issue," on page 71 for further information on determining pregnancy.

"If the extraction is being done at the time of an expected period, the uterus may not feel enlarged at all, even though the woman is in fact pregnant, but she may have some of the other signs of pregnancy: bloating, enlarged breasts, changes in appetite, nausea, and a change in the color of the cervix from pink to a purple or bluish cast," Emily notes.

SIGNS OF PREGNANCY

Objective Signs Missed period

Positive pregnancy test

Subjective Signs Nausea

Fatigue or sleepiness

Sensitivity to certain tastes or odors

Changes in appetite (cravings for certain foods, inability to eat certain others)

Weight gain

Breast tenderness

Breast enlargement

More frequent urination

Uterine Signs Softer uterus

Enlarged uterus

Cervical Signs Softer cervix

Change in coloration from pink to reddish, bluish,purplish

os more open than usual

ACKNOWLEDGEMENT OF
A WOMAN'S RESPONSIBILITY
IN MENSTRUAL EXTRACTION

"Long-standing, cohesive groups tend to have a good understanding among themselves about what menstrual extraction means, what it can and cannot do, and what the risks are," Adrienne says. "However, if a new member is having her first extraction, or if the group is doing an extraction for someone who is not a regular participant, it is very important that she clearly understands everything that will take place, and exactly what her role and responsibility in the process is."

"We've found discussions on this point to be very useful," Adrienne reports. "These discussions have been instrumental in our decision not to do any extractions outside of the group unless there is a very compelling reason to do so. In this case, we sometimes ask the woman to read and sign a sort of acknowledgment that she is familiar with menstrual extraction and is aware of the risks involved. We also go over our backup plan, so she knows what to expect if she needs to see a doctor or go to the emergency room."

CHECKLIST FOR MENSTRUAL EXTRACTION

"Quite a lot of supplies are needed for a menstrual extraction," Gabriella points out. "At each meeting one person assembles all of the accessory items and checks to see that we have what we need. Another person will go over the check list and a third will test the Del-Em™ to make sure it is working." (Possible sources of supply are listed on page 248).

Experienced self-helpers may not need to be prompted about the steps to a safe and successful procedure, but women who are training or those who do not do extractions very often may find a comprehensive checklist very helpful.

MENSTRUAL EXTRACTION CHECKLIST*

➡ Test Del-Em™ suction with cannula in a glass of water to make sure that suction is adequate and two-way valve is attached correctly.
➡ Make sure all equipment is disinfected.
➡ Speculums
➡ Flashlight with extra batteries (alt.: goose neck lamp)
➡ Plastic calibrated sound
➡ O-ring forceps, cervical stabilizer (Allis or single-tooth tenaculum) (alt.: kitchen tongs or long-handle tweezers)
➡ Rubber gloves (alt.: plastic wrap or plastic bags)
➡ Water-based lubricating jelly
➡ Tissues or paper towels
➡ Towels
➡ Gauze squares or cotton balls
➡ Sterile container
➡ Disinfectant
➡ Cotton swabs (long and short handled)
➡ Small dish or glass saucer
➡ Strainer
➡ Menstrual pads
➡ Written acknowledgement (if someone from outside of the group is having an extraction)

*This list represents a composite based on interviews with a number of self-help groups. For information on the Del-Em™ see page 241.

STERILE TECHNIQUE

"Knowing sterile technique is one of the essential keys to doing safe menstrual extractions," Emily notes. "There is a difference between instruments being *sterile*, being *disinfected*, and just being *antiseptically clean*. We found general agreement among experts that for procedures such as menstrual extraction and catheterization of the bladder, where there is no cutting involved and the vascular system is not invaded, 'high level disinfecting,' which kills most disease producing or infectious organisms, is sufficient."

"For menstrual extraction, sterile technique means getting the cannula, the only instrument to enter the body, thoroughly disinfected and making sure it does not touch anything once it is removed from its protective envelope or disinfecting bath before it enters the uterus," Gabriella

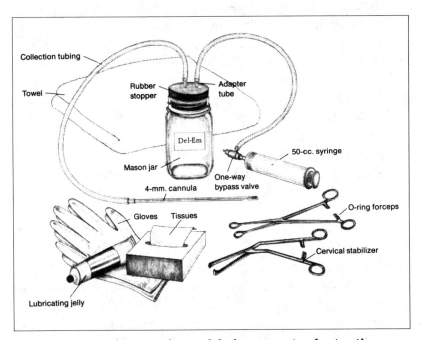

THE DEL-EM™ **and accessories used during a menstrual extraction.**

says. "Other instruments that touch the body should be thoroughly disinfected as well, to reduce the possibility of precipitating any sort of infection. The Del-Em™ doesn't need to be disinfected, though, since other than the cannula, nothing touches the vagina, cervix, or uterus." Gabriella notes that by virtue of having an opening to the outside of the body, i.e., the cervical canal, the uterus is not, strictly speaking, a sterile cavity. "It contains the same micro-organisms that exist in the vagina, but in such small quantities that they don't do any harm."

Groups without access to medical sterilizing equipment report that they disinfect their utensils for about 20 minutes with a number of over-the-counter cold sterilants including, among others, household bleach, povidone-iodine, and Zephiran. Gabriella notes that other solutions such as Cidex, Control III, and Septisol have been used effectively, but suggests that the manufacturer's labels be carefully studied before use.

According to Adrienne, "Povidone-iodine (Betadine, 7.5% or 10% solution) is also considered to be an excellent antiseptic disinfectant, killing all types of bacteria, yeasts, viruses, and protozoa." Up until about 1980, Zephiran was widely used in hospitals as a high-level disinfectant. However, it was discovered to be potentially toxic to newborns, and its use in the U.S. was generally discontinued in favor of other chemical sterilants. This problem notwithstanding, Zephiran, which kills most bacteria in about 20 minutes, is still marketed in the United States and is used in other countries.

"We've found that pressure cookers are an excellent way to disinfect metal instruments in a very short time—but you can't put cannulas in them," Emily says. "We also know groups that boil metal instruments in other types of metal containers with tight-fitting covers, or bake them in a hot oven." She points out that unless gauze or cotton balls (which are really *rayon* these days) are purchased sterile, they will contaminate things that have already been disinfected.

"Tap and bottled water are not sterile and will contaminate any disinfected instruments that are rinsed in them," Gabriella says. She also notes that bacteria will eventually grow in commercially produced "sterile" water, so it may be no better than tap water. "Freshly *boiled* water is definitely safe."

FOLLOW-UP

"We've found that conscientious follow-up is essential in staying on top of potential problems," Gabriella explains. "We stay in contact with each other every single day for about five days after an extraction, then every other day for a few more days. Because we are all friends, we tend to be in contact pretty frequently anyway. Normally, a designated member of the group will call the woman who had the extraction for the first few days, asking her how she is feeling, if she has been checking her temperature regularly, and how much bleeding she is having. If she thought she had been pregnant, she's asked if the signs of pregnancy have begun to disappear. Every woman who has an extraction watches carefully for signs of a complication, and if she notices *anything at all unusual*, she calls one of us immediately. The things we look for are severe cramping or abdominal pain, heavy bleeding or clots, and fever."

If signs of pregnancy do not begin to disappear within 10 days, the woman who had the extraction and two or more group members meet again, do uterine size checks to see if the uterus feels somewhat enlarged, and based on their findings, decide whether or not a reaspiration is in order. Whatever is extracted from the uterus during the reaspiration is carefully examined for chorionic villi—a sign that the extraction was not complete.

"If we don't see any villi, we begin to consider the possibility of a tubal (ectopic) pregnancy," Gabriella says. "We would then suggest that the woman see her own doctor for a blood pregnancy test and a sonogram."

POSSIBLE PROBLEMS

Because the technique for menstrual extraction is so similar to that of early termination suction abortion, similar problems can occur (see pages 221-239 for in-depth discussion of abortion complications).

Adrienne says that the most common problem with ME is the possibility of retained tissue if the woman having the extraction was pregnant. "We follow the CDC (Centers for Disease Control) guidelines: *When in doubt, reaspirate.*" The rate of reaspirations varies greatly from group to group, depending upon how the technique is practiced. One group that has been going for nearly 10 years estimates that its reaspiration rate might be as high as 20%.

Other groups have reported that they rarely have to reaspirate. Gabriella, whose group falls into this category, attributes their high completion rate to the use of a blunt-nosed "atraumatic" tenaculum or stabilizer, which looks something like a forceps. One end grips or pinches a place on the cervix, and the handle locks in that position. "If the uterus is retroverted (sort of curved or bent), it is often hard to get at an implantation that is in the top part or dome, called the *fundus*. Using a stabilizer allows you to tug on the uterus and straighten it out and get to the implantation easier," Gabriella explains. "We found out that in countries where menstrual regulation is done, reaspiration is often not feasible, so a tenaculum is routinely used to help reduce the chances of tissue retention. Some practitioners who have worked in clinics abroad have reported a very low rate of incomplete MR when they use a tenaculum."

"When reaspirating, we examine whatever we get very thoroughly," Gabriella says. "We noticed that once in a while, we got some rather large, pretty dense masses of tissue about the size and shape of bite-size candy—not like the feathery chorionic villi. We learned that this is retained tissue that the uterine lining, or developing placenta, has actually encapsulated. It's usually too big to be sucked through the cannula, so if the woman doesn't pass it on her own, she may need a suction abortion with a larger cannula or perhaps even a D&C."

Reports of uterine infections occurring in conjunction with a menstrual extraction are very rare. Adrienne's group had one infection in 100 menstrual extractions—a 1% infection rate. Indeed, none of the groups we surveyed had an incidence higher than 3%, which is comparable with the rate of infections for clinical abortions. "Conscientious daily monitoring is key to picking up infections right away and treating them before they become entrenched," Emily says.

CPR TRAINING

Self-help groups have found that menstrual extraction, like early termination suction abortion, has very few risks. Nevertheless, because the procedure can be slightly stressful to a woman's system, many groups feel very strongly that at least one or more people in the group know CPR (cardiopulmonary resuscitation). In fact, many women who do ME already have this training because of a strong interest in self-care. "All seven members of my group took the course together," says Adrienne. "We go through the routines every once in a while, to make sure everybody is on her toes."

A BACKUP PLAN

Every group we interviewed had a clear and easily executed backup plan that can be activated in case medical care or emergency advice is needed. Many groups have an informal arrangement with a sympathetic doctor, nurse, midwife, or other practitioner, who is willing to examine a woman if a problem develops, and who might be willing to arrange further medical care, including pregnancy termination, if necessary.

Occasionally, however, even a good backup plan can go awry. Doctors go out of town, nurses change jobs, and midwives can have very busy schedules. In this case, a self-help group has to be resourceful and tenacious. If no sympathetic practitioner is available, a trip to the emergency room is probably the next best choice.

Emily says that in six years, her group has had occasion to visit the emergency room once. "Someone developed a high fever that didn't go away after we did a reaspiration. We got worried. The doctor we would normally have consulted was away at a conference, so we decided to take her to the emergency room. I went with her and asked if I could stay with her during the examination. She told the doctor that she had a positive home pregnancy test, and was having waves of cramping, nausea, faintness, dizziness, and periodic bleeding, which at the moment had subsided. Just to make sure the doctor got the message, I asked the doctor if he thought that she was having a miscarriage. He felt her uterus and said he thought that she had already had it. He ordered routine urine and blood tests and discovered, much to our surprise, that she had a raging bladder infection that was not related to the menstrual extraction!"

Emily feels that "in an emergency room situation, or with an unknown practitioner, it is important not to give out more information than is necessary to determine that a miscarriage is occurring—for the legal protection of both the doctor and the woman who had the extraction, and for the group as well."

There are no known reports of a perforation from a menstrual extraction, but this does not mean that it couldn't happen. Gabriella notes that if it appeared probable that a perforation had occurred, her group has decided that they would—in that instance—tell the attending physician about the menstrual extraction. "You want to do everything you can to protect the woman's health," she says. "In a situation like that, only one of us would accompany the woman, so as not to expose the rest of the group if the doctor wasn't sympathetic to our situation."

Adrienne says that if after a second reaspiration the group has any question as to whether menstrual extraction is complete or if an infection has developed, they would not hesitate to seek medical advice. In any event, it's not easy for a doctor to tell whether you had an abortion, diagnostic uterine aspiration, or a menstrual extraction, especially the latter two, where the *os* is barely dilated. Emily observes that the only exception to this would be if a tenaculum was used and it left a noticeable mark on the cervix. "The marks usually disappear within a couple of days, or fade so much that they just look like a cervical blemish."

SECURITY PRECAUTIONS

Because menstrual extraction is a home health-care technique, it is not likely to be attacked in the way that abortion has been. Nonetheless, every self-help group needs to be aware of the potential concerns of friends, medical personnel, and even civic authorities about the legality of menstrual extraction. (See Chapter 8, The Legality of Menstrual Extraction.)

"Cohesive friendship groups are based on equal participation and trust, and probably don't have much to worry about in terms of being exposed to legal problems," says Gabriella. Nonetheless, anti-abortion zealots would like nothing better than to infiltrate a group, hoping perhaps to bring a legal challenge. To guard against this potential problem, many groups, like Gabriella's, "just don't let anyone into the group who doesn't have strong recommendations and a certifiable history of being pro-choice. I'd say that someone else in the movement has got to know them. Otherwise, we would tell them to start their own group."

Adrienne says that her group is "relaxed but watchful," being careful what they talk about on the telephone or in public places. She says that in her group and in several others she knows of, the training process provides ample time for members to get to know new members and get a good sense of their backgrounds, work situations, and social circles. "By the time they start doing actual menstrual extractions, we know them pretty well."

"I would think that the women in any self-help group might want to research their state laws regarding self-care and abortion, just to see what the parameters are," Adrienne adds. "That may sound unnecessary, but it's important to know what potential risks you are facing."

Many of the groups we interviewed have exacting policies about what they will do in case a problem arises. The policies are designed to protect both the group as a whole and the individual member. These policies tend to assume heightened importance in groups that occasionally do an extraction for someone outside of the group.

ARE FEARS ABOUT MENSTRUAL EXTRACTION JUSTIFIED?

While some doctors and family planning experts endorse menstrual extraction, others have expressed concern that while it is quite possible for paramedics and trained lay practitioners to do them responsibly, ME and other home health-care techniques might be misused by young women who are desperate and inexperienced, harming themselves in some way. But the scenario of young women harming themselves with menstrual extraction is based on an a lack of understanding of exactly what ME entails.

While the ME technique is elegantly simple, and many women have demonstrated that it can be learned by virtually anyone with a commitment to acquire such knowledge and skills, it is not something one can just decide to do. Menstrual extraction is a multistep process that requires considerable forethought, commitment, preparation, resourcefulness, and training over an extensive period of time. Acquiring information, becoming familiar with the reproductive anatomy, and assembling the equipment and learning to use it effectively are actually part of a months-long process. Realistically, there are enough stumbling blocks to discourage all but the most determined and resourceful women.

CHAPTER SEVEN

Two Menstrual Extractions

FOR THIS chapter, we visited a self-help group meeting and observed a menstrual extraction, and interviewed a woman who had an extraction when she suspected she was pregnant.

The scene is a modest bungalow on a palm-lined street in suburban Los Angeles. Tonight is the regular meeting of a self-help group that has been going on for about three years. Six women are expected: Amelia, Lauren, Zarela, Maxine, Robin, and Celia. Lauren has agreed to have her period extracted so that Zarela, the newest member of the group, can observe.

Amelia describes how a meeting begins:

"Our membership vacillates between eight or nine women and not everybody comes to every meeting." By 7:30 in the evening, all six women have arrived. Refreshments, which consist of sodas, tortilla chips and home-made salsa, are served, and the women chat for about 15 minutes. "We just like to talk a bit and get focused on who-ever is having an extraction," Amelia says. "Then we get down to the business at hand."

"My cycle varies from 28 to 35 days," Lauren says, "and today is day 33. I got my period about 8:00 this morning."

While Celia gathers up supplies and equipment brought by various people, the others explain the group's routines to Zarela. Celia will go over a checklist of critical supplies, set up the Del-Em™ and test it to make sure that the valve is attached and functioning properly. Then she scrubs and boils the O-ring forceps and blunt-nosed tenaculum, used to stabilize the cervix if necessary.

" I definitely had intercourse, so I guess my cervical cap worked," Lauren says. She is married and has a three-year-old daughter. For birth control she relies on a combination of fertility awareness and the cervical cap. "I use my cap about half of my cycle—up until I'm sure I've ovulated," she explains, "then I don't use anything until my period is finished. "We do want another baby, so I'm not so uptight about getting pregnant, but right now would be pretty inconvenient. I'm up for a promotion at work, and I don't want to blow it."

At this point, the group moves into the bedroom where Lauren takes off her pants and underwear and reclines on the bed with her back against soft pillows cov-

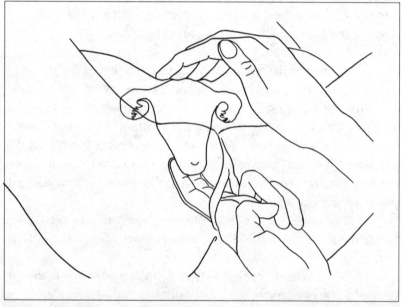

TO DO A UTERINE size check (also called a bi-manual exam), the examiner places the index and middle fingers of one hand into the vagina, and presses firmly on the cervix. The fingers of the other hand press on the abdomen, cupping the top of the uterus. The size of the uterus can then be compared to a chart like the one on page 155.

ered in African print fabrics. Amelia, Zarela, Maxine and Robin don latex surgical gloves and by turns assess the size of Lauren's uterus, just as they would if she thought she might be pregnant. They all agree that the size feels

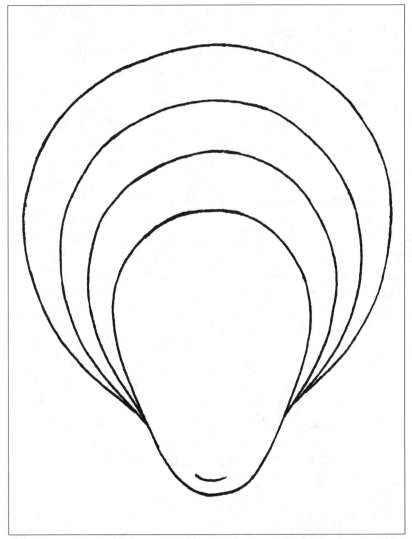

THIS CHART SHOWS the actual size of a non-pregnant uterus, and the uterus at various stages of pregnancy up to 12 weeks from the last menstrual period.

normal, i.e., non-pregnant, as they expected. Next, Lauren expertly inserts a plastic speculum into her vagina, and Amelia hands her a mirror and a flashlight. The speculum will stay in place until the procedure is over.

"It looks pretty pink to me," Lauren remarks. "Just like usual." In turn, Amelia, Zarela, Maxine and Robin hold the flashlight and peer intently into Lauren's vagina. "In my experience, you don't usually see distinct color change until about five to six weeks from the last period," Lauren adds.

Lauren gives the nod to go ahead with the extraction.

It has been decided that Amelia will be Lauren's "advocate" during the procedure. She will hold her hand, give her a sip of water or juice if she wants, and continually monitor her responses. Maxine will pump the syringe that creates a vacuum inside of the Del-Em™ and Robin will insert and manipulate the cannula. Celia will bring supplies as needed and massage Lauren's abdomen, legs, and feet if she has strong cramps.

"Let's get going," Robin suggests. "It's almost 8:30." Amelia sits on the bed beside Lauren, and Maxine gets the Del-Em™ from the table. Amelia asks Lauren if she is ready. "Yes," Lauren replies. "Ready to get rid of my period."

"You'll be eating pizza before you know it," Robin promises. "In the meantime, close your eyes, relax, and think of mozzarella." Everybody laughs, and then, as if by an unspoken signal, a reverential hush falls over the group. They feel, Celia notes in a whisper, that what they are about to do is significant, just a little bit subversive, and very powerful.

Using the O-ring forceps, Robin picks up some cotton balls that have been soaking in povidone-iodine, swabs out Lauren's vagina, and scrubs the cervix and the area around it vigorously. Then, again with the O-rings, she picks a 4mm cannula from an enamel pan where it has been soaking in Zephiran. Grasping its bottom with a gloved hand, she inserts it into the open end of tubing that is already connected to the Del-Em™ jar, and works at this until she is satisfied that the connection is secure.

This done, she says to Lauren, "I'm going to insert the cannula now."

"Okay," Lauren replies, taking a series of deep breaths.

The 4mm cannula is smaller in diameter than a pencil and exceedingly flexible. Holding it at a spot near its middle, Robin slowly and carefully guides its notched tip to the opening of the cervical canal about four inches from the entrance to Lauren's vagina. The tip slowly disappears into Lauren's cervix. "I'm at the inner *os* now," Robin indicates. Lauren winces and lets out a deeply held breath.

"Yeah, you are," says Lauren. "I can really feel it when the cannula goes through." Robin notes that Lauren is feeling more intense pressure as the tip of the cannula

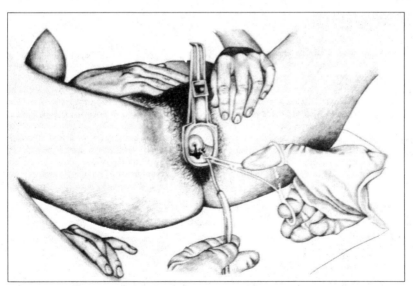

WITH HER RIGHT HAND, Robin is grasping the cannula with a pair of O-ring forceps, and is about to insert the tip of the cannula into Lauren's cervix.

presses against the tight band of muscle surrounding the inner opening, called the *inner os*, which protects the interior of the uterus from the outside world.

Amelia ask Lauren if she is experiencing any cramping. "On a scale of one to ten, I would say it's about a three," Lauren decides.

Things are a little bit tense now, especially for Lauren and Robin. Robin applies a little pressure and says, "I just felt the *inner os* give—the tip of the cannula is now inside the uterus."

Lauren lets out a sound that is a cross between a moan and a resonant "Ommmm." Amelia squeezes her hand and smoothes her hair comfortingly.

"That's right, stay focused on that mozzarella," Robin says, and she inserts the cannula in about another half inch. "I'm there," she announces, meaning that the tip of the cannula is touching the top or the *fundus* of the

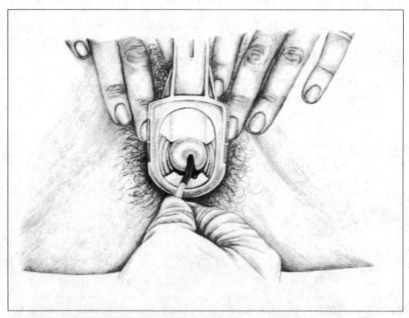

ROBIN HAS INSERTED the cannula into Lauren's cervix, and menstrual blood is beginning to be suctioned out.

uterus, sometimes referred to as the "back wall." She withdraws it a bit and says to everybody, "Can we start the suction now?" Maxine looks first at Lauren and then at Amelia. Lauren's eyes are closed and she is measuring her breathing. Amelia watches her for a few seconds, and deciding not to break her concentration, says softly, "Yes, go ahead."

Maxine begins to pump the syringe...three... four... five times. Lauren's brow furrows, her eyes are closed tight, and she lets out a long "Hummm."

"Cramping?" Amelia asks her.

"Umhunnnnnnnnh."

"I think it's a five," Amelia guesses.

The inside of the non-pregnant uterus is about three inches in length, and increases about an inch every month as a pregnancy progresses. Robin begins to move the cannula back and forth, withdrawing about one-half inch and then pushing in again. Now, she stops the back-and-forth motion and begins to rotate the cannula slowly. When she is finished, she will have rotated it 360° and moved it back and forth several times to cover the entire uterine interior.

About three minutes after the suction is started, blood appears first in the visible portion of the cannula shaft, and then in the clear plastic tubing, which is about twice the size of the cannula's circumference.

Lauren's eyes are now open and she looks at Robin. "Are you getting anything yet?"

"Yep, just now," Robin replies, with just a little note of triumph in her voice. "About three inches into the tube."

"How are the cramps?" Amelia asks Lauren solicitously.

"More, but not so bad. I've had worse during a period."

By now the extraction has been in progress about six or seven minutes, and blood has progressed about eight inches down the tube. Robin asks Maxine to pump again, and she presses again on the plunger.

Lauren has closed her eyes again and slowly rolls her head from side to side, as if to relieve tension in her neck. Amelia drops Lauren's hand and moves backward a bit, putting one arm under Lauren's neck in order to massage her muscles. After about five minutes of massage, Lauren winces visibly, and Amelia asks, "Do you want to take a break?" Lauren nods and everyone seems to let their breath out at the same time. Maxine puts the syringe down, but the cannula remains in place. As if recess has just been called, everyone except Lauren stands up, shakes, stretches, and walks around the room. Then a general assessment begins. Robin lifts up the tube and shines the flashlight on it, carefully inspecting it. If Lauren were pregnant, by now they would be seeing bright red blood mixed with the pale-yellowish chorionic villi, the characteristic tissue of the developing placenta. When rinsed and placed in a bowl with water, villi floats and appears feathery.

In about five minutes, Amelia asks Lauren how she is feeling, and when Lauren says fine, suggests resuming. Maxine does a few short strokes on the syringe, Robin moves the cannula back and forth, and the blood in the tube moves again, passing the halfway mark someone has placed on the tube. Sometimes during period extractions, blood only partially fills the tube and little or none drips into the jar. At other times, if a woman happened to be pregnant, the jar would partially fill with blood, blood clots, and chorionic villi.

Celia now takes a turn at the cannula. For three or four minutes silence reigns as she concentrates on the cannula, which she has now rotated all the way around so that the inch-long red mark on the cannula which ends just where the shaft disappears into the cervical *os*, has come full circle. Lauren groans and Robin asks her if she would like to have uterine massage. "Yes, that might be nice," she replies as she lets her breath out. Robin leans forward and places the fingers of both hands on Lauren's abdomen, pressing down in slow, kneading motion.

The actual extraction time has been about 15 minutes, and by now the movement of blood in the tube progresses only infinitesimally. "I think we're about through," Celia observes. "It's beginning to feel pretty rough." She asks Robin to take the cannula again and check. As she does, Robin explains, "When the uterus is filled with blood, its walls feel smooth and the cannula moves easily. As the uterus empties, it contracts, which the woman usually experiences as strong, sometimes painful cramping, and the walls become rough." Robin compares the feel of the cannula now to how it might feel if rubbed across a heavy towel. She confirms that the cannula is now difficult to move at all and that the uterine walls feel rough.

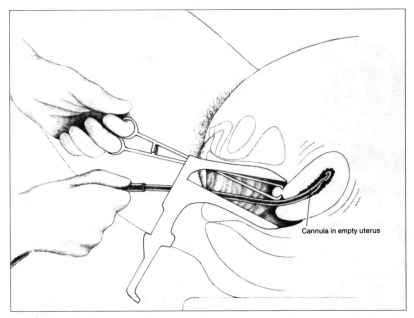

Cannula in empty uterus

THE WALLS OF the empty uterus have contracted around the cannula. Robin finds the cannula difficult to move, and the walls feel rough.

"Lauren, shall we call it quits?" Robin asks.

"Fine," she replies. "I'm beginning to feel pretty crampy."

Robin slowly withdraws the cannula from the cervical canal, and when the tip emerges from the vaginal opening, a collective cheer arises and tension evaporates as the group breaks into excited chatter. Lauren closes her eyes and takes several deep breaths. Amelia asks her how she's feeling and if she wants water or juice. She nods, and Amelia hands her a glass of apple juice. They sit quietly and talk while clean-up begins.

Celia gathers up the equipment and stores it in various gym bags and in a box to be left at Amelia's apartment. Maxine disconnects the syringe and takes the tubing and bottle of the Del-Em™ into the bathroom. She holds a strainer over a clear glass bowl, pours the contents of the jar through it, just as she would if the group had suspected that Lauren were pregnant. After washing the tubing and hanging it over a towel rack to dry, Maxine goes back into the bedroom to show it to Lauren.

"I don't see anything but blood," she reports. The others inspect it and agree, and Celia returns to the bathroom and empties the contents of the bowl into the sink. "That's that," she remarks and turns on the tap."

"Are you up for pizza?" Zarela asks. "I'll order."

"I think so," Lauren says brightly. "I really am hungry."

Amelia hands Lauren her underwear and pants, and she slowly gets dressed. They all go into the living room, where Lauren lies on the floor and does exercises designed to relax the pelvic muscles until the pizza comes Then the group sits down to enjoy a well-earned meal.

Marianne had her first menstrual extraction in 1986. She was not in a group at the time, but her friend Louise had been in one for several years. There was no abortion clinic in her town, so when she noticed signs of pregnancy, Marianne asked Louise if she knew where she could get an abortion. "Louise told me about a women's clinic in town a couple of hours away, but then asked me if I would consider having a menstrual extraction. At first I was a little skeptical, but after we talked for a while, I realized that my hesitation was based on things I had imagined that weren't true, and I decided to try it," Marianne says.

At the time, Marianne's period was about five days late. Louise called her group and they met at her house the next night. "We had a pretty long meeting before the procedure," Marianne remembers. "They showed me the equipment while they were testing it, and that made me feel more confident that things would go okay. Then we discussed the backup plan. If anything happened, we would call the clinic and someone would drive me there. I looked at my cervix with a light and mirror, which I had done before, and then Louise and two other members of

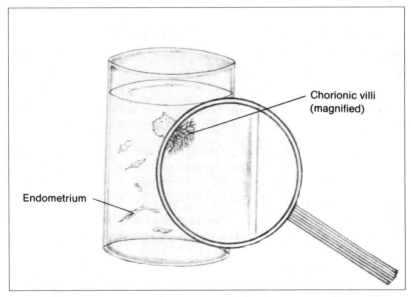

CHORIONIC VILLI, the placental tissue, is feathery and white, and floats in water.

the group felt my uterus. They thought it wasn't much enlarged, but that it felt softer than it normally would. Then I began to get a little excited that we were going to actually do it. Louise put the cannula at the entrance to my cervix, and then slowly pushed it into the uterus. I felt some mild cramping, which increased a little when the suction started. I was watching the cannula with a mirror and saw some blood coming into the tube. In just a couple of minutes we began to notice light-colored tissue mixed in with the blood. Ten minutes later, my cramps got stronger, but were not unbearable. After 15 more minutes, Louise suggested that we examine the tissue that had collected in the tube and jar. When we examined it, we saw a lot of chorionic villi and the sac, the membrane that contained the implantation. I felt relief, and all those things that women normally feel afterward, but I was also thrilled. I realized that I had complete control over my body, control I didn't have an hour ago, right there in my friend's living room! Needless to say, I joined the group."

These two accounts illustrate two experiences with menstrual extraction. Whether the extraction lasts 20 minutes, an hour, or longer, the vast majority of procedures are completed without incident, although, as Marianne observes, "They are all interesting, and a little bit different in some way.

"Menstrual extraction will probably never be practiced by that many women," she adds. "Learning it is a very serious and demanding project. But I think that every woman who is pro-choice would want to know about its existence, and know that she and her friends could learn it if they suddenly found themselves without any other safe options."

A NOTE TO THE READER

Women who do menstrual extraction consider it and other home health-care techniques to be completely legal, since an individual woman or a group of women cannot make a medical diagnosis of pregnancy; in fact, they are not attempting to do so. Therefore, they would not have the necessary intent required to consitute a criminal act of abortion. Also, women we interviewed maintain that they have the legal right to employ home-health care procedures, to drink teas or take vitamins to bring on a late period; or to extract the contents of the uterus with the help of family or friends. To our knowledge, menstrual extraction has never been judged to be illegal. Nevertheless, it is unpredictable what a court of law would decide in any given case, or what changes in the law will come about in future court decisions.

CHAPTER EIGHT

The Legality of Menstrual Extraction

OVER THE past 20 years, the excellent safety record of groups doing menstrual extraction has not presented the opportunity for a legal challenge, so its practice has remained in a gray area legally. Nevertheless, because of the potential for prosecution, many menstrual extraction groups have sought out attorneys and researched the laws of their states, in order to get a sense of the legal climate surrounding abortion and the use of home health-care techniques, and definitions of medical practice. This research, reviewed in this chapter, has raised some intriguing legal issues.

DIFFERENCES BETWEEN MENSTRUAL EXTRACTION AND EARLY TERMINATION SUCTION ABORTION

"We see menstrual extraction as very different from abortion," says Rosalind, who was among the first wave of women who learned the technique in the early 1970s. "While it definitely has the potential for terminating a pregnancy, as it is practiced menstrual extraction is so much more than that. Women who practice ME operate in a mutually supportive and mutually consensual environment, with the common goal of maintaining reproductive control. If a woman is worried that her period won't come, she can get it. If she doesn't want her period, for a variety of reasons, she can get rid of it. The assumptions upon which menstrual extraction is based are quite different than those of abortion."

Following is a list of factors Rosalind and other women we interviewed mentioned that differentiate menstrual extraction from abortion:

➡ Menstrual extraction is practiced at home by groups of lay women, while abortion is done by a doctor in an office or hospital setting.

➡ Menstrual extraction is usually done on or about the first day of the expected period, a time at which few women have *objective* evidence, i.e., information from a urine test, blood test, or a doctor's exam, that they are pregnant. In an abortion, pregnancy has been definitively diagnosed, and the intention of both the practitioner and the woman is to terminate the pregnancy.

➡ Small, close-knit groups of women learn menstrual extraction by reading, apprenticing to others who know the procedure, and by practicing on each other. This training is actually far more thorough than what most doctors are given in medical school. Doctors themselves usually learn to do abortions by working in an abortion clinic or by practicing on their own patients after doing a few procedures in their medical training or under the guidance of another doctor.

➡ Menstrual extraction is a process in which the woman receiving the extraction is an equal participant in the event. Abortion, on the other hand, is a service that is done for a woman, and money changes hands.

➡ In menstrual extraction, the suction used to extract the contents of the uterus is generated by pumping a large plastic syringe, while in the standard abortion procedure, the suction is created by a mechanical device called an aspirator.

➡ The instruments used in menstrual extraction are smaller and more flexible than in the standard suction abortion technique or in a D&C procedure. Consequently, less dilation of the cervical canal is required, causing less discomfort to the woman undergoing the procedure. In addition, chances of uterine perforation are less when smaller, more flexible instruments are used.

➡ A woman typically experiences far less discomfort during a menstrual extraction than during a standard abortion, but the procedure takes longer—about 15 minutes to one hour, compared to two to five minutes in the standard abortion procedure.

➡ Drugs are not routinely used in a menstrual extraction, whereas several drugs—usually unnecessary—are typically employed in an abortion. These drugs include a pre-procedure tranquilizer, an injection of anesthetic into the cervix to make dilation easier, a post-procedure drug to make the uterus contract to lessen bleeding, and prophylactic antibiotics to lessen the chances of infection.

Some of the differences in the two procedures are pronounced and others are subtle, but they strongly support the concept that menstrual extraction, as it is practiced, and abortion, as it is defined by law, are really quite different.

SIMILARITIES BETWEEN MENSTRUAL EXTRACTION AND THE INTRAUTERINE DEVICE (IUD)

"When a woman has a menstrual extraction she intends to get her period on or about the day she expects it, just as a woman who uses an IUD intends to get hers," says Rosalind. "This intent is very different from that of a woman who seeks an abortion and intends to terminate a known pregnancy. We see ME as similar to using a IUD." Rosalind sees the lack of such intent as critical to the IUD's status as a method of contraception rather than as an abortifacient.

Comparing menstrual extraction to IUDs may seem confusing at first, but they have more in common than is

immediately apparent. How IUDs actually prevent pregnancy is not well understood, but it has been suggested
that a foreign body in the uterus either creates a low-grade
inflammation or increases the production of
prostaglandins, or perhaps both, making the uterus hostile to the passage of sperm or to an implantation. It has
also been proposed that an IUD may somehow dislodge the
blastocyst after it becomes attached to the uterine wall, or
perhaps that it negatively influences the production of hormones necessary for the maintenance of pregnancy. What
is certain is that all of these theoretical modes of action
occur well after the union of sperm and egg. As a matter of
fact, the time frame in which an IUD and menstrual
extraction work is essentially the same: in the majority of
cases, about two weeks after fertilization.

HOME HEALTH CARE TECHNIQUES

"Women who have done menstrual extraction for many
years see it as a home health-care technique, similar to
self-catheterization, bladder instillations, or giving oneself
an enema," says Alexis, whose self-help group has carefully researched the legal ramifications of menstrual
extraction. Alexis points out that medical supply houses
and drugstore shelves are filled with products such as eye
washes, ear syringes, blood pressure cuffs, home pregnancy tests, syringes for self-injection, and a host of other
over-the-counter drugs and devices that are intended for
routine health monitoring or maintenance.

"With minimal training, people can perform these
home health-care procedures themselves, or with the aid
of family members or friends," Alexis says. "Women can
now identify and treat yeast infections, people with AIDS
may start their own IVs at home, people with painful

bladder inflammations are learning to instill anti-inflammatory solutions directly into their bladders. In fact, children as young as eight years old who have severe bladder dysfunction are taught to catheterize themselves." Alexis observes that these home health-care techniques are known to have minimal risk and are safe enough to be done without the supervision of or sometimes even the advice of a physician.

AN HISTORICAL PERSPECTIVE ON ABORTION LAWS AND HOME HEALTH-CARE TECHNIQUES

From Colonial times to the early 19th century, abortion was widely practiced but unregulated in the United States. The first restrictive laws, enacted in the 1820s and 1830s, were passed not to keep women pregnant, but to keep them from dying.[1] Later, from the 1840s through the 1880s, there were less humanitarian reasons for the regulation of abortion. According to a fascinating "friends of the court" brief filed in 1991 by 250 American historians in support of Planned Parenthood in *Planned Parenthood of Southeastern Pennsylvania v. Casey*, these reasons included "...the medical profession's desire to control the practice of medicine, openly discriminatory ideas of the appropriate role for women, opposition to non-procreative sexual activity and to the dissemination of information concerning birth control, and even concern for racial and ethnic purity."[2] A number of respected studies of the history of abortion laws have noted that the prime impetus behind restrictive laws was organized medicine's desire to corral the profits from the lucrative abortion trade.[3,4,5,6,7]

HOME HEALTH-CARE TECHNIQUES: Up through the second decade of the 19th century, about the same time that the earliest laws regulating abortion were enacted, healing in the United States was done primarily by female lay practitioners who relied on knowledge of European folk medicine brought to the New World by the Colonists, and on the rich Native American lore. In the 1979 feminist classic *For Her Own Good*, Barbara Ehrenreich and Dierdre English note that the campaign of so-called "regular" physicians to control medical practice, which was initiated in the 1830s, provoked a mass reaction that culminated in the formation of a widespread and active "Popular Health Movement." At the same time, spurred by the nascent women's movement, women began to take a renewed interest in their own health care. "From swapping medical horror stories, women's circles moved on to swap-

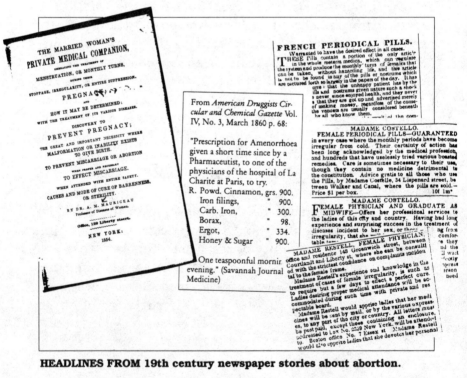

From *American Druggists Circular and Chemical Gazette* Vol. IV, No. 3, March 1860 p. 68:

"Prescription for Amenorrhoea given a short time since by a Pharmaceutist, to one of the physicians of the hospital of La Charite at Paris, to try.
R. Powd. Cinnamon, grs. 900.
Iron filings, " 900.
Carb. Iron, " 300.
Borax, " 98.
Ergot, " 334.
Honey & Sugar " 900.

One teaspoonful mornir evening." (Savannah Journal Medicine)

HEADLINES FROM 19th century newspaper stories about abortion.

ping their own home remedies, and from there to seeking more systematic ways to build their knowledge and skills. There were 'Ladies' Physiological Societies,' where women gathered in privacy to learn about female anatomy and functioning—something like the 'know-your-body' courses offered by the women's movement today."[8]

Up through the 1920s, and in rural areas up through the Great Depression of the 1930s, people relied on doctors for life-threatening situations, taking care of more routine health matters themselves using herbs, over-the-counter remedies, and common sense.

In the last quarter of the 20th century, social history has come full circle. In the 1970s, interest in natural foods, alternative healing techniques, and self-care increased explosively, and the modern women's health movement, which focused primarily on reproductive health issues, was born. The phenomenal popularity of *Our Bodies, Ourselves*[9] opened the gates for a flood of women's self-help literature, which quickly spilled over into every area of medical care. Women's health activists focused on abortion, the lack of safe contraceptive options, high cesarean rates and dangerous childbirth practices, unnecessary hysterectomies, breast cancer, menopause, the misuse of hormone replacement therapy, and other crucial issues. In the 1980s, allied with other activists and consumer groups, this movement broadened its interests to include AIDS, sexual abuse, safety in the workplace, and a host of other social and medical concerns. In the 1990s, in the face of a crumbling health-care system, the insurance crisis, and the all-out attack on women's right to safe abortion, the concepts of alternative healing, self-help, and home health care are taking on a new and compelling resonance.

Today, even the tradition-encrusted idea that only doctors can do abortions safely is also beginning to crumble. Since 1976, 20% of all abortions in Vermont have been performed by Physicians Assistants, and their safety record is as good as that of physicians themselves. Because of the severe shortage of doctors willing to do abortions, there is also a growing movement to permit Nurse Practitioners to do abortions in the first trimester of pregnancy. In the developing world, the use of menstrual regulation [see pages 123-127], a technique nearly identical to menstrual extraction, has demonstrated that lay people can perform such procedures safely.

CONSULTING AN ATTORNEY

Even though menstrual extraction has been practiced safely for many years, its proponents recognize that they do run a small but irreducible risk of legal prosecution. If such a challenge is made, it is likely to result from someone being injured—slightly or seriously—during an extraction. Prosecution will probably be made under current abortion laws, as well as under laws governing the practice of medicine.

Even though good legal arguments can be made that doing a menstrual extraction is not practicing medicine, and that legally, it is not an abortion, certain prosecutors may be anti-abortion and on the lookout for the opportunity to bring a suit. Even prosecutors who are pro-choice may believe that the technique is too dangerous to be practiced safely by lay people and feel compelled to take a case. Jurors may harbor such sentiments as well.

Because of the volatile atmosphere surrounding abortion and women's rights to control their own reproduction, menstrual extraction groups have increasingly sought counsel to help them research the laws of their specific states, to help them ascertain how they can work safely within those laws, and to assess, as far as possible, the chances of prosecution under existing laws. **In doing** legal research, women in various self-help groups noted the following issues and questions as being particularly relevant:

➡ **definitions of critical terms such as "diagnosis," "treatment," or "condition."** For example, does a mother recognizing that her child has a sore throat constitute a "diagnosis"? Does giving a family member an aspirin constitute "treatment"? Are menstruation and pregnancy defined as pathological, i.e., abnormal, conditions?

➡ **the definition of "medical practice."** Most laws define "practicing medicine" as holding oneself out as being able, and offering, to diagnose, treat, operate, or prescribe. Typically, legal cases have involved unlicensed practitioners holding themselves out to the public as being "experts." Thus far these laws have not been applied to the ministrations of one family member to another. Women in menstrual extraction groups note that they are not holding themselves out as experts. Instead, they maintain, each member of the group is aware of the training and capabilities of the other members, and all members are equal participants. Would current definitions of medical practice apply to this mutually acknowledged arrangement?

➡ **regulations governing home health care.** What types of procedures are commonly done at home, and how are they regulated? For example, could a person be prosecuted for instilling an anti-inflammatory solution into his or her bladder without a doctor's order?

➡ **vagueness of statutory language,** which might result in the law being enforced in a capricious or oppressive manner, and a literal interpretation of the law producing absurdities.

➡ **can the law withstand a constitutional challenge?** That is, does the law violate rights guaranteed by the Constitution such as free speech, freedom of assembly, or the right to privacy? The right to privacy, guaranteed by the

Constitution, is the underlying principle of *Roe v. Wade*. Under *Roe*, states must show a compelling interest regulating abortion. It is unclear how far states can go in regulating activities that are done, within the privacy of a self-help group, by its members, to control their own bodies and physiological processes. Today, many old anti-abortion laws might be ruled unconstitutional because they interfere with constitutional rights.

➡ **legal precedents that might be applied to menstrual extraction.** Since menstrual extraction has never been challenged legally, there are no factual precedents.

➡ **established exceptions to relevant statutes.** Most laws are written in fairly general terms; therefore, exceptions can almost always be found.

➡ **conspiracy issues such as "facilitating," "aiding and abetting," or "covering up" something considered to be a crime.** In efforts to win a conviction, prosecutors may attempt to bring charges of conspiracy, but whether such charges can be upheld depends upon whether or not menstrual extraction itself is judged to be a crime.

➡ **intent.** In order to be prosecuted for a crime, a person must intend to break a law. Many statutes require only a general intent, i.e., if a person can be shown to have engaged in forbidden acts, then they are guilty. Other statutes require that the person have a "guilty mind" and to have intended to commit a crime. In the United States, laws governing the practice of medicine usually require that only general intent be proved for conviction. Abortion laws, on the other hand, usually contain language indicating knowledge and willfulness. In a legal case involving menstrual extraction, a prosecutor would probably have to show a specific intent to cause a "miscarriage." But from the perspective of a woman having a menstrual extraction, she just wants to get her period, whether she is pregnant or not. She may suspect she is pregnant, and in fact, her whole group may suspect that she is pregnant, but by most state laws and by standards of medical practice, neither a woman or her group can make a medical diagnosis of pregnancy. At the early stage that most menstrual extractions are performed, only a blood test or chemical pregnancy test administered on the order of a doctor could definitively diagnose a pregnancy. Of course, when the extraction is finished, the group will look to see if tissue indicating the presence of a pregnancy has been extracted, and pregnancy may be retrospectively determined. But from the woman's point of view, the procedure was not an abortion, either medically or psychologically. From a legal perspective, a prosecutor would need to show, beyond a reasonable doubt, that a woman and her friends intended to do an abortion, as abortion is defined in the law of that specific state.

FINDING THE RIGHT ATTORNEY

Many attorneys consider it their job to advise their clients of the most conservative action, to "keep them out of trouble." Others attempt to help their clients navigate the murky and often shifting waters of the law, helping them to avoid potentially rocky shoals and treacherous currents. Many attorneys are "strict constructionists" and favor a literal interpretation of the law. Others adhere to the school of "legal realism" and see the law not as some fixed code, but rather, as a set of fluid, changing rules dependent upon how individual judges interpret them.

In seeking an attorney, menstrual extraction groups might be wise to evaluate their attorney's legal philosophy and, if possible, find one who is familiar with, or at least open to, the concept and philosophy of menstrual extraction. Then they can work to establish a mode of operation comfortable for everyone in the group.

WHO IS AT RISK FOR PROSECUTION?

In interviewing women in menstrual extraction groups, we talked to some whose activities were mostly or entirely limited to learning self-examination, researching basic health issues such as vaginal infections, discussing the philosophy of ME among themselves, and perhaps speaking publicly about it. Operating under the protective umbrella of free speech, these groups are not at much risk for prosecution, and could serve a valuable function by doing consciousness raising about menstrual extraction in their communities. And if a self-help group in their community were to be prosecuted, they could provide ready assistance in organizing a legal defense and community support.

Other groups focus not only on the philosophy of menstrual extraction, but learn the technique and practice their skills. Some groups may do extractions for themselves and, occasionally, for a close friend or family member of someone in the group. These groups may be at some risk for prosecution, but probably only if a serious complication occurs, and then only if someone outside of the group learns of the incident and takes action.

A few groups, however, say that if abortion becomes illegal or generally inaccessible in their states, they are prepared to seek ways to circumvent or defy local laws. These groups see their training as preparation for starting illegal abortion services, patterned after the activities of Jane (see pages 106-109) in the 1970s, as well as other lay abortion providers who operated before abortion was legalized. Groups that provide a service are operating in a different realm: they have the same obligations to the public as any licensed practitioner does and would face the same legal ramifications if a complication occurred.

Most menstrual extraction groups develop their philosophy over a period of many months, or even years, and find the mode of operation most comfortable for them.

"At first we were so energized by the possibilities of menstrual extraction that we wanted to do it for everybody," says Candida, who started a group in 1990. "At the beginning of the second year, our group split in two. A few women were committed to doing community MEs when it was convenient for them, but after we looked more closely at the state laws, most of us decided to limit our activities to just ourselves and our friends. We found this arrangement a lot less anxiety-producing." Candida notes, however, that if stringent anti-abortion laws were to be enacted in her state, "we know what to do, and we know how to do it."

CIVIL DISOBEDIENCE

Some of the women we interviewed, especially the ones who have done thorough legal analyses of their activities, have characterized the practice of menstrual extraction as a form of civil disobedience. This practice, as defined by Abe Fortas, a Justice of the Supreme Court from 1965-1969, involves willfully breaking what is perceived to be an unjust or unconstitutional law to bring public attention to a problem.

As it has come to be understood in the law, there are two basic types of civil disobedience. In one, there is a law against a certain type of activity, and a person or group of people knowingly break the law and do not attempt to evade punishment when they are arrested. For example, the Rev. Martin Luther King and other civil rights activists often marched without permits to protest racial discrimination, and when they were arrested, pleaded guilty and went to jail.

A few women we interviewed said they suspect menstrual extraction is illegal, but they do it anyway. Because they feel that they are breaking the law, they operate sub rosa and do everything they can to avoid official scrutiny.

In a second type of civil disobedience, some people may think laws on the books against certain activities are invalid, inapplicable, or unconstitutional, and therefore, they engage in the activity, believing that what they are doing is not a crime. For example, in India, Gandhi and his followers believed that the British tax on salt, considered a necessity for everyday life, was illegal, and challenged the law by making it themselves. The point was so obvious that they were not arrested, and this single act of civil disobedience became a powerful symbol of Indians' need to control their own destiny. Many women who do menstrual extraction do not believe it is illegal and may, in various ways, press for their right to practice it.

The proponents of this second type of civil disobedience choose to interpret the law in the broadest possible terms, and consequently, are constantly pushing the frontiers of social propriety, governmental regulation, the law, medicine, or whatever, in order to establish new standards of acceptability and enlarge the arena for human activity.

THE YOGURT DEFENSE

Most legal precedents in which lay people have been charged with practicing medicine without a license have involved unlicensed people rendering services which are useless, shoddy, dangerous, or are grossly misrepresented by advertising. Few cases involve women helping each other by mutual agreement in the promotion and maintenance of their own health care. There are two precedents, however, in which Carol Downer, the co-developer of menstrual extraction, was involved: these vividly illustrate the potential difficulties of prosecuting women who do menstrual extraction.

In 1972, Carol's self-help group was busted, and she and Colleen Wilson, another group member, were arrested. Colleen was charged with 10 counts of practicing medicine without a license (PMWL) including doing a menstrual extraction, fitting a diaphragm, giving a member a packet of birth control pills, and removing one of the member's tampons.

Colleen had pressing family responsibilities, and was about to be accredited as a teacher and did not want to put her license at risk, so she entered a plea bargain, pleading guilty to one count of PMWL: fitting a diaphragm. The other charges were dropped, and Colleen was given two years probation. Carol was charged with one count of PMWL: having inserted yogurt into the vagina of one of the group members as a treatment for an overgrowth of yeast. (In the early 1970s, women's anatomy and physiology was so mystified that the prosecutor thought that acts requiring a medical license had been performed.) Carol went to trial and was acquitted by the jury, which did not find treating a yeast condition with yogurt to be practicing medicine.

The outcome of this case illustrates how the concept of what constitutes the practice of medicine has changed, not because of a change in the law, but from a change in social ideas. Today no prosecutor would arrest a woman for inserting yogurt into a friend's vagina or helping her to remove a tampon, but 20 years ago they would, and did.

Four years later, in 1976, Carol and other lay health workers at the Los Angeles Feminist Women's Health Center were under investigation, and this time the charge was not just for the use of yogurt. A woman came into the clinic and asked for birth control pills, even though she had a health problem that was a contraindication to pill use. After a health worker explained the risks of taking birth control pills with such a condition, the woman insisted on taking them, and, reluctantly, the health worker gave them to her. The charge was practicing medicine without a license.

During a pre-trial conference, Carol remarked to the Deputy Attorney General that she did not consider the health worker's action to be practicing medicine.

"Well, Ms. Downer, how do you determine what constitutes the practice of medicine?" the Deputy Attorney General demanded.

Carol's attorney started to object to the question, but let her continue.

"First," Carol said, "we study the particular activity and evaluate which skills, training, and knowledge are required to perform it. Then we consider whether a lay person could safely perform that particular activity. If the answer is 'yes,' then we ask ourselves, 'If a lay health worker were to get arrested for this particular activity, and if the case were to go to trial, would the *jury* think that what we did constitutes practicing medicine without a license?" The Deputy City Attorney, who was to prosecute the case, was also present and listening intently. "If we think that a jury would decide that we were not practicing medicine without a license," Carol continued, "then we do it." The Deputy City Attorney shook his head, snapped his notebook closed, and said, "I have no intention in getting involved in *this* case. The matter is closed."

Of course, there are so many variables that no one can predict how any particular case might turn out. These cases illustrate, however, how careful legal preparation can influence the outcome of a case.

Times change, and the way the law is interpreted changes with it, and this process of ferment and change is as political as it is legal. Therefore, it is essential for women who are blazing new social trails to understand how political the legal process is, and to be highly conscious of existing law and of the social currents that swirl around it.

CHAPTER NINE

Herbs and Other Traditional Methods of Fertility Control

THE EARLIEST means of limiting family size were probably breastfeeding, which naturally suppresses fertility for a time; avoiding intercourse; or reduced fertility through the demands of vigorous work. When these methods failed, women relied on folk remedies to terminate unwanted pregnancies, using potions and aromatics, magical rituals invoking unseen forces, cervical irritation, hot baths, and uterine massage. Women in ancient cultures also appear to have had knowledge of herbs with estrogenic properties, which may have prevented ovulation or implantation, as well as an extensive pharmacopoeia of herbal abortifacients.[1] Desperate and uninformed women frequently resorted to douching with caustic substances, to physical abuse, and to a horrific assortment of uterine probes and washes. In spite of little scientific evidence that these methods work, all are still employed today. Some are patently useless, and others, while they might terminate a pregnancy, are so dangerous that they are as likely to maim or kill as they are to be effective. Nonetheless, salted away among this catalog of horrors are methods that have been used in the past to safely terminate unwanted pregnancies, and which may be used again as abortion becomes less accessible. For the most part these are methods of last resort.

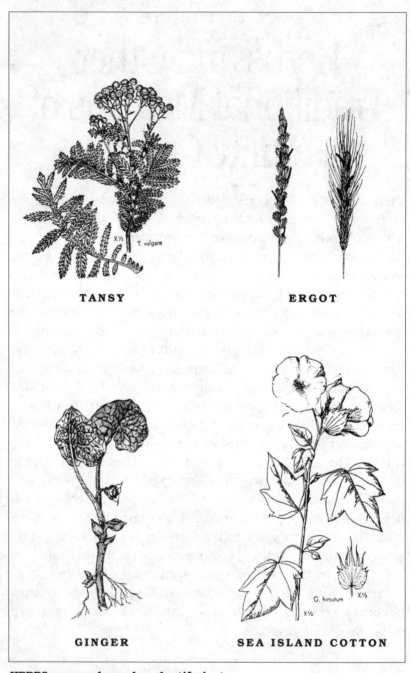

TANSY

ERGOT

GINGER

SEA ISLAND COTTON

HERBS commonly used as abortifacients.

HERBS

While herbs have been widely employed both as contraceptives and as abortifacients, there is little reliable data on their effectiveness, toxic levels, or possible effects upon the developing fetus. One difficulty in getting concrete information about herbs is that claims about their use and effectiveness are almost always anecdotal, but are often reported as fact, even though they have not been subjected to any accepted form of scientific scrutiny. It is difficult to determine the cause and effect relationship of herbal regimens to miscarriage, because there is seldom proof that the woman was pregnant to begin with, and because about one in six fertilizations ends in miscarriage anyway. For example, based on a few isolated reports, there has been some interest in investigating the possibility that wild carrot seeds (daucus carota), the seeds of Queen Anne's Lace, might prevent implantation of a fertilized egg,[2] but funding to do a study on a large enough sample of women is hard to come by.

Another problem in using herbs effectively is that herb books and alternative healing manuals tend to assume a good deal of knowledge on the part of the reader, and, perhaps effort to avoid the appearance of prescribing, these sources tend to be somewhat general and imprecise. Yet another problem in ascertaining the effectiveness of herbs as contraceptives or abortifacients is that the medical profession and drug companies have shown little interest in carrying out formal studies on anything except the most commercial preparations.

In spite of these problems, there are so many reports of success in inducing the menstrual flow and in precipitating miscarriage from herbalists and women all over the world that it is difficult to dismiss them all as mere coincidence.

HERBS SAID TO HAVE
ABORTIFACIENT PROPERTIES

Some herbal manuals note that certain herbs have abortifacient properties, but often such herbs are referred to as "menstrual inducers." Just like drugs, all herbs have certain actions, and most seem to have multiple actions, which can be confusing to the uninitiated. Most of the herbs said to promote menstruation or induce a miscarriage fall into one or more of these categories: abortifacients, herbs that cause miscarriage; emmenagogues, i.e., herbs that "promote menstruation," perhaps by stimulating contractions of the uterine muscle; oxytocic herbs, which imitate the action of the pituitary hormone, oxytocin in stimulating uterine contractions; stimulants, herbs that stimulate uterine contractions; and vasoconstrictors, which contract blood vessels, perhaps cutting off the fetal blood supply.

The herbs most frequently mentioned as having these properties are:

HERB	ACTION
angelica	emmenagogic, stimulant
black cohosh	emmenagogic, stimulant
blue cohosh	emmenagogic, oxytocic
celery	emmenagogic
cotton (seed or root)	abortifacient, emmenagogic, oxytocic
ergot	abortifacient, emmenagogic, oxytocic, vasoconstrictor
ginger	emmenagogic, stimulant
horseradish	stimulant
mistletoe	abortifacient

motherwort	emmenagogic
parsley	emmenagogic
pennyroyal	abortifacient, emmenagogic,
Peruvian bark	oxytocic
shepherd's purse	vasoconstrictor
tansy	abortifacient, emmenagogic

Numerous other herbs with similar or other actions have also been reported to be effective, but those most frequently mentioned as potential abortifacients are black and blue cohosh, pennyroyal tea (not pennyroyal oil), and tansy, often used in combination with each other and with other herbs. These herbs may be the most effective, but they can also be toxic and may even cause death in extreme cases. Herbalists warn women with high blood pressure to use vasoconstrictors with extreme caution, since they may increase blood pressure.

SOME PRECAUTIONS WHEN USING HERBS

Before attempting to bring on a menstrual period using herbs, it would be useful to check information in standard herbal books (see Suggested Reading, page 259), or to consult a reliable herbalist who might be willing to share his or her information about effectiveness and risks.

Many herbs, like many prescription drugs, can be toxic when taken in large doses or when taken over a long period of time. In 1978, a woman in Denver, apparently thinking that she was pregnant, died a slow and painful death from taking a high dose of pennyroyal oil.[3] The woman lived for seven days after she took one ounce of pennyroyal oil, suffering two heart attacks, liver and kidney failure, and disseminated vascular coagulation (see pages 233-234). Since this incident, health practitioners and herbalists have been adamant that pennyroyal oil not be used in trying to bring on a menstrual period or precipitate a miscarriage. Others have noted that this is an extremely isolated case, and that other preparations using pennyroyal tea have been used safely, and sometimes successfully, by thousands of women to bring on a late period. In any event, it is clearly unwise to exceed the recommended dosage.

When using herbs, herbalists recommend watching carefully for signs of toxicity such as nausea, vomiting, sweating, chills, fever, headache, ringing in ears, dizziness, low blood pressure, difficulty in swallowing, extreme thirst, diarrhea, rapid pulse or heartbeat, muscle spasms, restlessness, drowsiness, unusual talkativeness, fatigue, and tremor. Herbalists cite more dramatic symptoms of toxicity including hallucinations, mania, collapsing, convulsions, and coma. If any of these symptoms occur, go to an emergency room and/or consult a doctor immediately or consult your state or local poison control center, which is often listed in a prominent place in telephone directories.

Some herbalists point out that if bleeding has not commenced after having missed a second period, or after having taken an herb at the recommended dosage for two weeks, it seems useless and perhaps dangerous to continue. Prolonged ingestion of some herbs may cause nerve damage or other negative effects and may cause fetal abnormalities if the pregnancy is carried to term.

EXPERIENCES OF WOMEN USING HERBS TO INDUCE MENSTRUAL FLOW

One of the most convincing published reports of success in inducing a miscarriage with herbs is Deborah Maia's intimate diary, *Self-Ritual for Invoking Release of Spirit Life in the Womb: A Personal Treatise on Ritual Herbal Abortion.* (See Suggested Reading, page 259). This 24-page pamphlet consists of a diary Maia kept for 17 days beginning five days after her expected menstrual period, during which she drank herbal preparations, took hot baths, visualized herself aborting, and engaged in personal spiritual rituals.

Deborah had a positive home pregnancy test, and according to her diary, it seems likely that the herbs she took did precipitate her miscarriage. Initially she took fresh ginger root tea for five days, then switched to a combination of blue cohosh, black cohosh, and rue, in tincture form (distilled herbal essences in an alcohol base). On the fifth day of her regimen, she assessed her situation and her commitment, and evaluated her options—to have a clinical abortion or to carry her pregnancy to term—if a second round of stronger herbs didn't work.

Although the herbs apparently worked, it is possible that they might not have if Deborah had not been so in tune with her body rhythms and so psychologically focused on ending her pregnancy; her experience clearly illustrates the fact that there is considerably more involved in bringing on a late period or precipitating a miscarriage herbally than just sipping herb tea and waiting a few days. It may involve an unwavering commitment of two weeks or more, with no guarantee of success in the end. Whether or not one is spiritually inclined, Maia's book is essential reading for anyone who is seriously interested in pursuing herbal remedies for birth control or pregnancy termination.

Herb lore and advice on mixtures, doses, and formulations vary widely from book to book and among herbalists themselves, so women who are considering using herbs for fertility control might be wise to check information in standard herb manuals and to consult a reputable herbalist as well.

VITAMIN C

Vitamin C plays a vital role in collagen formation and cell repair, and has been touted as a cure for everything from the common cold to cancer. In the mid-1970s, reports of an article by E.P. Samborskaia in a Russian scientific journal created a stir of interest in the use of this vitamin as a potential abortifacient.[4] In this study, which is not known to have been duplicated, 20 pregnant women took about six grams of ascorbic acid (a synthetic form of Vitamin C) for three days, and all but four had started to menstruate by the end of the three days. The author of this study believed that high levels of Vitamin C stimulated the increase of estrogen and precipitated miscarriage.

In spite of the unduplicated claims of articles such as this, many women have used Vitamin C as an abortifacient and seem to think it works best if doses of up to six grams a day are initiated a few days before the expected period and continued for five to seven days. There is also a general agreement among herbalists that initiating this regimen several days after the expected period yields less reliable results than beginning beforehand, and in fact may not work at all.

High doses of Vitamin C are thought to be harmless in general, except that they can promote the formation of crystals in the urine and possibly urinary stones, if taken over a very long period. Therefore, some experts on vitamins suggest that women who have kidney problems avoid taking high doses of Vitamin C over a prolonged period of time.

OTHER METHODS OF
PRECIPITATING A MISCARRIAGE

Historically, as a method of last resort, cervical irritation has been one of the most widely employed types of abortion. This method does not require much in the way of equipment or skill, and because nothing enters the uterus, it does not appear to be dangerous in the way that coat hangers or knitting needles are. Moreover, it can be done under the most adverse and desperate circumstances. Essentially, this method involves using a finger or long handled cotton swab to dilate the cervical canal and/or stimulate cervical nerves, which in turn may stimulate uterine contractions. When successful, cervical irritation can sometimes induce a miscarriage, while other times it simply brings on some preliminary symptoms, and a woman may then have to seek a medical termination of her pregnancy, if available.

DIGITAL IRRITATION

The Abortion Handbook (see pages 104-106), describes the digital (meaning "finger") variation of cervical irritation, noting, "Nowhere is there even a man-made law that says a woman can't put her very own finger into her very own uterine canal or vaginal tract." The authors caution women to cut their nails and scrub their hands vigorously before beginning:

> *This uterine stretching business is a slow process, sometimes taking up to six weeks of daily effort (say twice per day), and well may not work at all...The miscarriage will not start immediately with a gush of blood...Hopefully, the contractions will start up, feeling like menstrual cramps. They*

should increase in intensity like small labor pains, and eventually, you might expel the embryonic debris (fetus) after the first few weeks of applying the finger method. This expulsion will be in the same manner as a massive menstrual period, complete with tissue and heavy blood clots.

Toby, a therapist who has practiced in New York City for many years, reports her experience with cervical irritation in the mid-1940s:

My first abortion was a D&C done by a doctor in his office on the Upper West Side. It was brief and not traumatic, but it was very painful. The next time I got pregnant, I was upset because I was supposed to leave for Europe the following week. Frantic, I asked a psychoanalyst I knew if he knew anyone who did abortions, and he gave me the name of a man who had helped many of his patients. I called the man and he came to my mother's apartment the following day. He told me that he had gone to medical school in Boston, and that during that time had worked for a doctor who did illegal abortions. He said that he later went to Sweden and learned the digital method which was much safer and less painful. He didn't use any instruments. I lay on the couch and he put his finger in my vagina to "irritate the nerves in the cervix" for a few minutes. Nothing happened, but I guess I expected it to at some point, so at the end of the week I sailed for Europe as planned. By the time the boat docked in France, I felt very pregnant and didn't know what to do, but I couldn't envision finding a doctor who spoke English, let alone one who would do an abortion, so after a few days of agonizing, decided to return home and took the next available boat. When I arrived, I called and told him I was still pregnant, and he said that it was not unusual to have to do the procedure twice. Again, he irritated my cervix for a few minutes, and told me that he was sure it would work. It certainly did. The next day, I had cramps somewhat stronger than my usual period, and in the evening, I expelled a fetus about an inch and a half long into the toilet.

Toby was lucky. Instead of back alleys, seedy hotel rooms, or riding around blindfolded, she had the support of her mother and was able to get a reliable referral for a safe, respectful abortion. Many women in her situation had to endure enormous health risks, financial exploitation, and some were subject to sexual exploitation as well. Women who must seek underground abortion services need to be aware that they are especially vulnerable and need to be prepared to defend themselves. See page 13 for information on costs of an abortion, and page 34 for self-defense against sexual harassment.

One of the most poignant reports of digital irritation abortion that we came across was from a doctor who was a prisoner in a Nazi concentration camp during the Second World War. Interviewed in a 1982 British Broadcasting Company (BBC) documentary on Holocaust survivors, the doctor said that pregnant women in his compound were taken away for medical experiments, and when they were taken for that purpose, they never came back. He reported doing cervical irritations with his finger, causing many miscarriages to occur, and thus saving numerous women's lives. "My fingers were filthy," he said, "but no one ever got an infection."

Stories such as this one are emblematic of how important information on safe, non-clinical methods of pregnancy termination can be. In addition, millions of women whose circumstances are not so nearly as dramatic or life-threatening have been deeply grateful for information on simple home procedures that can safely interrupt a pregnancy when no doctor is available, willing or legally allowed to do an abortion.

CATHETERS

Catheters, slim, flexible rubber tubes, are routinely used in medical procedures to infuse or to drain fluids (such as urine), from the body, Since the 1940s, and possibly much earlier, catheters have also been used by doctors and by women themselves to precipitate miscarriages. Doctors often inserted catheters in their offices and instructed women to return after several days to have them removed, or to remove them at home themselves. Sometimes the vagina was packed with cotton to hold the catheter in place. The tip of the catheter was inserted one to two inches into the uterine cavity and remained in place for several days, serving as an irritant to stimulate the uterus to contract.

Olivia, a midwife who served a rural area of Wisconsin in the 1960s and 1970s, relates her experience using catheters to start miscarriages.

I learned to insert catheters from an older general practitioner who worked in this area for over 30 years. The main difficulty I found was that very small catheters are as flimsy as cooked spaghetti, and at first I had a hard time getting the tip through the cervical canal. The doctor taught me to put the small catheter inside of a larger, firmer one, and then, after the tip is inside the uterus, to withdraw the larger one. He also taught me to pack the vagina tightly with gauze to help keep the catheter in place. The catheter tip serves as an irritant, and the uterus begins contracting almost immediately to try to reject it. Spotting usually starts within a day or two, and cramping increases. If a miscarriage didn't occur within five days, I would remove it and do intensive uterine massage. This would usually increase both cramping and bleeding, and the woman could then go to a doctor and complain of smyptoms of a miscarriage. In my experience, the incidence of incomplete miscarriages was quite high, and infection was very common too. After all, a catheter is an open tube that provides a freeway for traveling bacteria. The doctor told me that he had seen a number of women die from unattended catheter-induced infections, and encouraged me to monitor women closely for several weeks afterward.

Dr. Alex Brickler's account of treating the complications of illegal abortions, on page 100, underscores how dangerous catheters can be if they are used improperly and without access to medical back-up.

LAMINARIA

Sticks of sterilized compressed seaweed, called laminaria, are routinely used in second trimester abortions to dilate the cervix more slowly, gently, and safely than can be done with metal dilators. In addition to the traditional sticks of compressed seaweed, there is now a synthetic type of laminaria called Dilapan. Both the seaweed and the plastic sticks are a little longer than the average cervical canal, and when they are inserted the tip may actually protrude into the uterine cavity. Therefore, there is always some risk of infection.

Practitioners who do later abortions have observed that occasionally a woman who has laminaria in place will go into active labor and deliver the fetus at home, before her abortion appointment. Therefore, clinics that use laminaria advise women that the dilation of the cervical canal effectively starts an abortion and that if they change their minds about having an abortion after insertion, they may not be able to carry the pregnancy to term. Women are also cautioned that because the pregnancy is interrupted, they are at risk for infection if the laminaria are left in place longer than the prescribed time, or if the pregnancy is not then terminated. Because the laminaria go into the cervical canal, they need to be inserted by a doctor, midwife, or other trained technician who is knowledgeable about women's anatomy and has worked with someone who is skilled in laminaria insertion.

In the past, sticks of the inner bark of slippery elm were sometimes inserted into the cervical canal and would expand over a couple of days in a way that is similar to laminaria. Over about two to five days the bark would expand to several times its normal size, dilating the cervical canal and acting as an irritant, causing cramping, bleeding and uterine contractions. Infection was probably exceedingly common with slippery elm bark because it could not be adequately disinfected.

UTERINE LAVAGE

Uterine lavage ("washing") has long been employed as a method of self-abortion, using a rubber ear syringe or catheter to infuse a liquid substance into the uterus. This is one of the more dangerous methods of self-abortion that have been employed by desperate women, primarily because of the assumption that the stronger the solution, the higher the success rate. Unfortunately, this bit of folk wisdom is dead wrong. Many women have suffered severe injury or have died from infusing all manner of caustic substances—quinine, lye, kerosene, bleach—into the vagina (not knowing where the uterine opening is), or into the uterus itself. Another risky aspect of uterine lavage is the possibility of introducing air into the uterus and causing an air embolism (an air bubble that gets into the blood stream and causes death if it reaches the heart).

In spite of these significant risks, uterine lavage has been done safely. Doctors, midwives, and others have long known that infusing a sterile saline solution into the uterus will precipitate a miscarriage. In skilled, caring hands, it appears that uterine lavage can be done safely, but it has the same disadvantages that hospital saline procedures have: the procedure takes a lot longer than an D&E and is emotionally more traumatic, because women have to go through actual labor and then deliver a dead but relatively large fetus.

DRUGS

MORNING-AFTER PILL: The probability of pregnancy resulting from a single incidence of unprotected intercourse is estimated to be less than 20%, so if any unprotected intercourse occurs, there is not necessarily a reason to panic. However, because of the unavailability of abortion care, parental notification requirements, imminent travel plans, or a host of personal reasons, some women find the time until pregnancy can be confirmed to be unendurable. In these cases, if unprotected intercourse occurs, the so-called morning-after pill may be a reasonable option.

The morning-after pill used to be a five-day regimen of DES (diethylstilbestrol), a powerful synthetic hormone that was widely used in the past as a long-term injectable birth control drug, to suppress lactation, and as a treatment for the signs of menopause.[5] Although DES is not FDA-approved for use as a morning-after pill, it was widely used in the past for this purpose, and some doctors still prescribe it. However, because of unresolved questions about the safety of DES, many doctors, clinics, and college health services instead prescribe two mega-doses of Ovral, a birth-control pill that contains both synthetic proges- terone and high doses of synthetic estrogen. (This use of Ovral is not approved either, but clinicians seem to have less concern about this pill than about DES).

To be effective, two doses of Ovral must be taken 12 hours apart, starting no later than 76 hours after an inci- dent of unprotected intercourse; the closer to the time of exposure to sperm, the better. If taken in the prescribed fashion, the Ovral morning-after pill appears to be about 98% effective in interrupting the normal flow of events just after fertilization.

Ovral is a high-dose birth control pill and has some of the same undesirable physical effects, whether you take it for contraception or as a preemptive abortifacient. Although this is a one-time dose, women who have high blood pressure or are at risk for strokes or heart attacks should use this method with caution.

Katrina, a graduate student in Denver, found that taking the morning-after pill wasn't necessarily an innocuous experience. "I only took it once, and wouldn't care to do it again," she says. "After the first dose, I was so nauseated that I didn't want to take the second one, but I really didn't want to get pregnant right then, and it was available from the student health service for free, so I did. Luckily, it was at night, so I just went to bed, and was so sick and dizzy that I couldn't move." Katrina notes that she did get her period, right on time.

Not everyone who takes the morning-after pill suf- fers such negative effects. Kozue, a drama student in New York City, says that she took both doses of Ovral with a dose of anti-nausea medication—and performed in a play that night. "The worst time was just before I went on, and it was probably exacerbated by pre-performance anxiety," she says. "But once I got into my part, my adrenalin kicked in and I completely forgot about feeling lousy."

The morning-after pill is no substitute for reliable contraception. At $50 or more a pop, it is expensive if used repeatedly, and, as the experiences of Katrina and Kozue illustrate, its effects can range from disagreeable to temporarily incapacitating. In addition, the long-term risks of taking such high doses of synthetic hormones are not known. Yet women who can find a clinic that provides morning-after contraception may, on occasion, be able to avoid the greater inconvenience of having an abortion. This method of fertility-intervention is especially useful in cases of rape or incest if there is any chance that a pregnancy might result. Women who report rapes within three days and go to a doctor or emergency room for an examination often ask to take the morning-after pill rather than wait and see if a pregnancy results.

PROSTAGLANDINS: Prostaglandins are substances manufactured in the body from fatty acids and, among other effects, cause powerful contractions of the uterine muscle during labor. Synthetic prostaglandins have been used to do abortions (a single injection causes miscarriage in a high percentage of cases), to help control bleeding after later abortions, and to increase the effectiveness of RU-486 (see page 207). Because of a high incidence of disagreeable and sometimes violent ill effects, and because better procedures, i.e., the D&E procedure (see pages 89-91 and 230-231), were developed, prostaglandin-only abortions were never employed in the United States. Prostaglandins are still commonly used in Europe for abortions, perhaps because many doctors have not learned to do D&Es.

CYTOTEC: In developing countries where abortion is illegal or generally unavailable, women usually start their abortions by any means at hand, then go to a hospital where they can have the abortion completed. For the most part, these methods are unsafe and the results are frequently disastrous. Recently, however, a report from the Brazilian state of Ceara revealed that many women were taking Cytotec (*misoprostol*), a prostaglandin-like drug that is used to lessen the impact of anti-inflammatory drugs on the gastrointestinal tract, to start miscarriages. Most women took four or more 200-microgram tablets for several days, or inserted them into their vaginas, using them as a suppository. In the manufacturer's studies of Cytotec,[6] the drug caused miscarriage in 11 percent of women, and precipitated uterine bleeding in an additional 41 percent. People who take Cytotec regularly as an anti-ulcer medication may experience disagreeable effects such as diarrhea, abdominal pain, headache, nausea, and constipation, and such problems may occur on a short-term basis as well.

A report in the British medical journal *The Lancet* expressed grave concern about misuse of Cytotec for starting a miscarriage especially about incomplete miscarriages, and the potential for fetal malformations if miscarriage did not occur. The report noted, however, that post-miscarriage complications, especially infection, were lower "than with any other drugs or procedures used to induce abortion."[7]

Most prostaglandins are given as an injection, except for Cytotec, which comes in pill form, and *gemeprost*, a prostaglandin suppository made by the Japanese company Ono. The suppositories have been used in France, England, and in World Health Organization studies to increase the effectiveness of RU-486.

While herbal menstrual inducers and abortifacients, and other traditional methods of pregnancy termination are not as reliably effective as clinical abortion, when used appropriately and with care, they can be safer than the methods covered in Chapter 10, "Folk Methods That Are Dangerous and Don't Work." Ideally, if the onslaught of anti-abortion legislation can be stemmed, these methods will never again be necessary on a large scale, and will quietly collect dust on the shelf of historical curiosities.

CHAPTER TEN

Folk Remedies That Are Dangerous and Don't Work

HISTORICALLY, information about unsafe methods of terminating pregnancies has been more widely available than information about safe, effective methods, causing millions of women to endure serious and often permanent injuries or to suffer painful and untimely deaths. Following is a compilation of methods that desperate women have used when they had no information about safer self-abortion techniques, or when they had no safe options available.

Knitting needles, coat hangers, sticks, wires, etc. Everyone has heard about abortions being started with knitting needles or coat hangers and the disastrous, often deadly results. In *The Abortion Handbook*[1], Lana Phelan and Pat Maginnis warn, "All knitting needles should be marked by the manufacturer, 'This object may be hazardous to health if used for abortion purposes.'" They note ironically that most often when such instruments are used, the uterus is punctured, causing the woman injury or death; but the fetus, in many instances, remains unharmed.

Caustic substances such as soap, bleach, quinine, lye, kerosene, castor oil, etc. Many women who aren't very familiar with their reproductive anatomy often believe that drinking or douching with noxious substances will damage the fetus and precipitate a miscarriage. But because the placenta encapsulates the fetus in a self-contained system, these methods generally only harm the woman, causing severe, perhaps irreparable damage to the delicate mucous membranes of the throat, stomach, or vagina. While infusing caustic substances into the uterus with an ear syringe or catheter might interrupt the pregnancy, they may kill the woman in the process. In particular, uterine infusions may introduce air into the uterus which can then enter the blood stream (air embolism) and cause sudden death.

Physical abuse such as a fall from a high place, hitting the abdomen, jogging, gymnastics, horseback riding, or other such jarring activity may precipitate a miscarriage, but the likelihood of success is low, except, perhaps, fairly late in pregnancy. In that case, there is the high likelihood of delivering a live, but very frail fetus. Some women actually go so far as to abuse themselves physically, or have their partner or friend do it, and often end up in the emergency room to have their wounds bandaged, and are still pregnant. The uterus is a tough, muscular organ that evolution brilliantly constructed to protect the growing fetus from such insults. From all reports, women who engage in strenuous activities such as jogging, gymnastics, or horseback riding, are far more likely to wind up with sore muscles than they are with a miscarriage.

Wendy, a 16-year-old high school student in Philadelphia, tried to start her own miscarriage.

> *I drank some brandy straight and took some pills a friend got for me, and when I was good and high, I rolled down the stairs, hoping to knock the pregnancy loose. What actually happened was*

that I got a lump on my head and chipped a ver-
tebra in my back, but I still didn't get my period.
After that, I wasted a lot of time taking every drug
I could get my hands on, but nothing worked. By
the time I went to a clinic, I was 14 weeks preg-
nant, and the abortion cost $400. I couldn't get the
$100, so I had to tell my father. He was furious,
but gave me the money, and afterward, he
restricted my activities for six months. Now I can't
go out even on weekends, and my back hurts all
the time.

Hot baths. It is known that hot baths will cause harm to a developing fetus, but there is no evidence that it will reliably start a miscarriage. Fatigue, burns, and possibly painful scarring are the only predictable results of this method. Theresa, a 15-year-old high-school student in the Bronx, New York, reports that after she sat in scalding hot water for several hours, her burns were so bad that she had difficulty in walking for more than a week. She remained pregnant.

Street drugs such as alcohol, marijuana, crack cocaine, heroin, LSD, mescaline, or PCP (angel dust), etc. Rumors always seem to circulate around high-school locker rooms that taking lots of whatever drugs are available will kill a developing fetus and/or cause a miscarriage. All of these so-called recreational drugs, and even a lot of prescription drugs, are highly toxic and may cause nausea, vomiting, fainting, and other disagreeable effects (see symptoms of toxicity on page 188), but they are more likely to harm the fetus than cause an abortion. In cases of alcohol abuse, the fetus may be born with *fetal alcohol syndrome*, which can result in severe developmental and behavioral problems.

Not eating. Women sometimes try to get rid of a pregnancy by eating and drinking very little. Starving does deprive the fetus of nutrition and may ultimately damage it in numerous ways, but the major damage is to the mother, whose body begins to digest its own muscles and other tissue in order to support the fetus. In addition, if a woman decides to carry a pregnancy to term after a period of severe starvation, the fetus is at very high risk for physical and developmental difficulties, and the mother may suffer lifelong problems as well.

Prayer. There is no evidence that prayer will keep a woman from getting pregnant or that it will help cause a miscarriage.

GETTING HELP

History is littered with the bodies of women who, out of sheer desperation and a lack of information, attempted to end their pregnancies with the only means they could think of—sharp instruments, harsh substances, physical abuse, or drugs. If women are injured or die trying to abort unwanted pregnancies because safe, legal facilities are outlawed, the blame rests not with them or with those trying to help them. It rests squarely on the shoulders of the religious right, on state legislatures that have passed regressive abortion restrictions, and on the U.S. Supreme Court, which has chosen to limit access to safe abortion facilities.

If you are desperate and can't tell a family member, friend, teacher, or someone else you trust, take a look at Chapter 2, "Information Networks," for information on how to find help. **If you are determined and persistent enough, someone will help you.**

CHAPTER ELEVEN

Is RU-486 the Wave of the Future?

THE FRENCH abortifacient drug, RU-486 *(mifepristone)*, is the first in a new category of drugs called *anti-progestins*, which among other actions, interfere with the production of progesterone, the hormone that supports and nurtures pregnancy. RU-486 blocks the production of progesterone in the uterus by competing with progesterone for receptor sites in cells in the uterine wall. Because there is more RU-486 than progesterone available (if you have taken the recommended dosage of 600 mgs.), it will fill a large number of the receptor sites, somewhat like a key fitting into a lock. Deprived of progesterone, the placenta will wither and disintegrate. If a pregnancy has recently been implanted on the uterine wall, it too will separate from the uterine wall and be expelled.

In order to be effective, RU-486 must be taken when a woman is five to seven weeks pregnant (seven to nine weeks from the last normal period). By itself, RU-486 is effective in terminating pregnancy about 80% of the time, but taken in conjunction with a "booster" of *prostaglandin* (PG), a hormone that causes the uterus to contract, the effectiveness increases to about 95 or 96%. *Cytotec*, an ulcer medication that is also in the prostaglandin family, has also been used as a booster. *Cytotec* appears to work as effectively as other prostaglandins do, and has slightly less severe side effects (see pages 199-200).[1]

Under the French protocol, a woman takes three 200 mg. tablets of RU-486 and goes home. In a few cases, this 600 mg. dose is enough to precipitate a miscarriage, which at this early stage is often similar to a heavy, crampy period. Two days later most women return to the clinic and take *Cytotec* or receive a prostaglandin suppository *(gemeprost)* in their vaginas. **About 95% of these women will have miscarriages within about four hours. In the other 5% of cases,**

➡ the blastocyst may separate from the uterine wall, but is not expelled because the uterus does not contract hard enough, or because the cervix does not open enough for the tissue to pass. In either case, the doctor or other technician can simply remove the tissue with small forceps; or
➡ the blastocyst does not separate at all, or does not do so completely, and the woman needs a standard suction abortion to complete the procedure.

On a metabolic level, the action of RU-type drugs is exceedingly complex, and at this early state of development, not entirely understood. So far, the possibility of fetal deformities, if a woman fails to miscarry and decides to carry the pregnancy to term, are unknown. (In contrast,

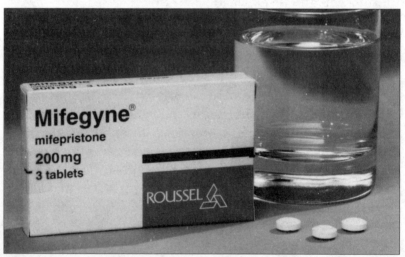

THREE 200 mg. tablets of RU-486, equaling 600 mg., packaged for use in England.

fetal deformities *are known* to occur with the use of Cytotec). Therefore, any woman who takes these drugs, fails to miscarry, and decides to continue her pregnancy, should be aware of the possibility of having a child with perhaps severe malformations or developmental problems.

PHYSICAL EFFECTS

Nearly all of the physical effects of RU-486 + PG abortions are attributable to the prostaglandin booster, and are generally similar to the effects of early termination suction abortion. **These are**

➡ cramping, ranging from moderate to severe and lasting for several hours until the miscarriage occurs. About 10% of women experience cramps severe enough to require pain killers.[2]

➡ bleeding, ranging from four to 40 days, with an average of about 10 days. About one woman in 1,000 receives a transfusion when blood loss is higher than acceptable levels.

➡ dizziness, nausea, vomiting, diarrhea, which occur in a small percentage of women. While they can be uncomfortable, they are transient and can usually be treated with medication.

PRACTICAL ADVANTAGES
AND DISADVANTAGES

As a method of abortion, RU-486 has some great practical advantages. Because no instruments enter the uterus in RU-486 procedures, the incident of infection is minimal, and there is no possibility for perforation of the uterus. In addition, doctors do not need special training to dispense RU-486 as they do in order to do competent suction procedures, so RU-486 abortions could potentially be provided on a much wider scale, making abortion more accessible.

The primary disadvantage of RU-486 abortions is that, as it is administered in France, it requires four visits. In the U.S., it could probably be provided in two visits, with an optional follow-up visit if necessary. RU-486 also requires medical supervision and follow-up, which may not always be available in developing countries.

AN RU-486 ABORTION

Danielle, a 28-year-old French women who had an RU-486 abortion in 1990, describes her experience:

One week after my initial exam, I stopped by the hospital on my way to work and a nurse gave me six pills, which I was required to take in her presence. I had some very faint cramps the next day, but nothing else happened. Two days later, I returned to the hospital at 9:00, along with four other women. We each got the prostaglandin injection and then sat in a room on couches and chairs. We were allowed to eat and drink, and we read magazines and talked to pass the time. Two of the other women's boyfriends came with them, and one brought her mother. The atmosphere was very calm. The nurse told us that we would feel cramps, and that soon they would get pretty strong. She said that when we felt stronger contractions and pressure in the vagina, we should go into the bathroom and sit on the toilet. Florence, one of the other women, went first. She came out looking perfectly normal and carrying a plastic pan, designed to fit under the toilet seat to catch the expulsion. About 11:30, just as the nurse predicted, I felt sort of hard camps, and definite pressure in my vagina, so I went to the bathroom and sat on the toilet. I would say that I had about seven or eight distinct contractions and felt something warm slip out of my vagina, and then I felt some blood coming out also. In two or three minutes, I looked in the pan and saw a little clump of tissue the size of a 10-franc piece [about the size of a quarter] and some blood clots. I took it to the nurse and watched while she washed it and checked to see if the abortion was complete. Mine came out whole and when it was washed, it looked like a little rubbery dumpling, nothing more. I had some cramping and period-like bleeding for seven or eight days, and then some spotting for another week, but I never experienced nausea or fatigue like some women do.

Danielle says that the RU-486 abortion was far different than the one she had in the hospital when she was 19 years old. "This time, I felt like I was in control, and taking the pills felt so much safer than having anesthesia and having some doctor poke at you with instruments."

A few women miscarry at home, before returning to get the PG injection, but they return to the clinic or hospital for an examination.

RISKS OF RU-486

Although RU-486 has not been as widely used as other methods of pregnancy termination, it has been studied extensively in France, England, and numerous other countries. As a result, it appears that RU-486 compares very well with other methods of abortion, especially early termination suction abortion, both in terms of short-range risks and of effectively terminating unwanted pregnancies.

From a medical standpoint, because no instruments enter the uterus, there is no chance for perforation, and because no anesthesia, not even a local anesthetic, is necessary, there is no risk of anesthesia-related complications. Uterine infection may occur if there is retained tissue, but so far this incidence has been exceedingly low. In France, if the abortion does not appear to be complete, the doctor does a suction procedure on the same day.

With RU-486, bleeding lasts an average of 10 days, but for a few women, it can last up to 40 days, which is slightly longer than for suction abortion. A few women, whose bleeding has been either more severe or longer lasting than normal, have received blood transfusions.

SERIOUS RISKS

Among the 110,000 women who have taken RU-486 thus far, there have been a tiny number of major problems: one woman had a mild heart attack, one had a stroke, and one woman died. All of these women smoked, and the first two were over 35 years of age. The woman who died was a heavy smoker, and was seeking to terminate her 13th pregnancy. This suggests that she may have been poor, and as a consequence, may have had multiple health problems.

After the first two serious incidents, RU-486 researchers decided to limit use of RU-486 to non-smokers under 35, but made an exception for the woman who died. Her death was extremely unfortunate, and probably would not have occurred if the guidelines had been strictly followed.

RU-486 is a steroid compound whose metabolic action is complex and not yet entirely understood. Since this drug, like the birth-control pill, has general metabolic effects that disrupt the reproductive process, as yet unknown effects are bound to surface when it is available for use on a wide scale in less affluent populations. Nevertheless, given the experience thus far, RU-486 appears to be about as safe as taking a dose of penicillin.

As it is given in France, RU-486 requires four visits, as compared to two for early termination suction abortion. The number of visits required for RU-486 is more comparable to those for standard second trimester abortions. An RU abortion also takes longer—about four hours from the time a woman takes the prostaglandin booster until the miscarriage is completed—as compared to one to two hours in the clinic and a three- to five- minute procedure for early termination suction abortion.

THE DEVELOPMENT AND MARKETING OF RU-486

T I M E   L I N E

1968   Hoechst, A.G., a German chemicals conglomerate,acquires an interest in Roussel Uclaf

1974   Hoechst, in second acquisition, acquires 54.6% interest in Roussel Uclaf

1980   RU-486 synthesized

Roussel Uclaf applies for patent for RU-486

1982   First human studies done with RU-486 in Switzerland

French government acquires 36% interest in Roussel Uclaf

1988   **June 23**—Roussel Board of Directors meeting at which opposition to RU-486 surfaces

Sept. 23—RU-486 approved in France

Oct. 24—RU-486 marketed in France

Oct. 24-25—Protest against RU-486 in France led by Catholic hierarchy

Oct. 26—Roussel Uclaf Board of Directors votes to withdraw RU-486 from market

Oct. 28—French Health Minister Claude Evin declares RU-486 "the moral property of women" and orders drug back to market

Nov. & Dec—Series of meetings between Roussel Uclaf & Hoechst regarding further marketing of RU-486

Nov. 21—First meeting of Reproductive Health Technologies Project, a task force of U.S. pro-choice activists, to promote public education about RU-486 and other anti-progestins

Dec. 15—Decision made not to distribute RU-486 outside of France

Dec. 27 or 28—RCR Alliance, U.S. anti-abortion group, delivers threatening "Declaration" to Hoechst headquarters in Frankfurt, demanding a meeting with Hoechst executives

1989   **Jan. 3**—Hoechst agrees to meeting with RCR Alliance, but no meeting ever occurs

1990   **July 24 & 25**—Fund for the Feminist Majority delegation meets with President of Roussel and with a committee at Hoechst

July—RU-486 becomes issue in California gubernatorial contest

June 27—AMA passes resolution supporting testing of RU-486

September—New York City Mayor David Dinkins announces support for RU-486

1991   **June 19**—U.S. State Department threatens to cut funding of World Health Organization if any U.S. funds are used in testing of RU-486

June 20—State Department softens opposition to RU-486

June—New Hampshire legislature passes bill HCR 11, calling for study of RU-486

July 1—RU-486 becomes available in England

Dec. 6-7—Conference on Anti-progestin Drugs: Ethical, Legal and Medical Issues, Arlington, Va., sponsored by American Society of Law & Medicine

1992   **Feb. 20**—Second Fund for the Feminist Majority delegation meets with Hoechst committee in Frankfort

WHY RU-486 IS NOT
MORE WIDELY AVAILABLE

The U.S. anti-abortion movement panicked when it first learned about RU-486, supposing that the drug would give "unrestricted access to abortion to every household in the entire world,"[3] but this anti-abortion nightmare is wildly overblown. Because of the need for medical backup with RU-type drugs, their use will probably always be restricted to clinic or hospital settings. Nonetheless, RU-486 would provide a safe and effective abortion option for many women.

The U.S. anti-abortion movement has been given lavish credit for keeping RU-486 off the U.S. market, but early on, advocates for RU-486 became aware of a more insidious and problematic obstacle to its distribution— opposition to abortion within Hoechst, the company that owns a controlling interest in the drug's French manufacturer, Roussell Uclaf, and to some extent, within Roussel itself.

Roussel has repeatedly cited threats of a boycott by anti-abortion forces as the primary reason for its failure to distribute the drug more widely. It is an open secret, however, that Dr. Wolfgang Hilger, the long-time Catholic Chairman of Hoechst, and many high management officials at Hoechst (and to a lesser extent at Roussel) are opposed to abortion. Even though Hilger's opposition to abortion was noted in *The New York Times Magazine*[4] and in a cover article on Roussel in *Pharmaceutical Executive*,[5] the media has focused entirely on boycott fears.

RU-486 was patented in 1973, one year before the German company Hoechst bought a controlling interest in Roussel-Uclaf. Hoechst did nothing to interfere with research on the drug until its marketing in France evoked a shrill public outcry instigated by France's Catholic archbishop, Jean-Marie Lustiger. Two days later, due to enormous pressure from Hoechst, and against the wishes of Dr. Edouard Sakiz, the president of Roussel, the Roussel Board of Directors, (which includes several Hoechst loyalists), voted to remove RU-486 from the market. But because the French government also owns one-third of Roussel's stock, the Health Minister, Claude Evin, forced Roussel to re-market RU-486, making his now legendary declaration that "RU-486 is the moral property of women."

ARE FEARS OF A BOYCOTT REALISTIC?

Roussel has repeatedly claimed that it has failed to apply for approval of RU-486 in the U.S. because of fears of a boycott by anti-abortion groups. And indeed, anti-abortion groups have threatened to attempt to boycott both the products of Roussel and Hoechst. However, Roussel distributes only a few prescription drugs through its parent company's U.S. subsidiary, Hoechst/Celenese. (Doctors, most of whom are pro-choice, would have to be the primary boycotters of prescription drugs.) For its part, Hoechst manufactures primarily agricultural and industrial chemicals and fibers, which are sold in bulk to wholesalers, who then distribute to manufacturers. Eventually, these products appear in manufactured goods such as carpets, tires, synthetic fabrics, cigarette filters and paints—and thus would be nearly impossible to identify.

The final nail in the boycott theory is the timing of the Hoechst/Roussel decision to severely limit distribution of RU-486. That decision appears to have been made firmly and finally before the first direct contact by the RCR Alliance and other U.S. anti-abortion groups. On December 27 or 28, 1988, the RCR Alliance delivered a 20-page "Declaration," threatening not only a possible boycott but other types of corporate terrorism to Hoechst's sprawling headquarters. This was nearly two weeks *after* a

December 15 board meeting at which Roussel, under intense pressure from Hoechst, decided not to market RU-486 outside of France.

To many family planning experts and pro-choice advocates who have followed the RU-486 controversy, it is clear that Hoechst does not want its name associated with abortion, especially in countries where abortion is very controversial. Putative fears about a boycott have perhaps served as a smoke screen which has conveniently masked behind-the-scenes machinations of powerful Hoechst board members and their allies at Roussel.

RU-486 was allowed to be marketed in England only after a protracted intra-company struggle and an act of Parliament amending the 1967 English Abortion Act to allow RU-type drugs to be dispensed in physicians' offices. English women will be able to receive RU-486 as a "day treatment," but foreigners are ineligible to receive RU-486 in England. This was apparently instituted at the request of Roussel Uclaf, to limit the drug's use to British nationals or residents only.

Because of Hoechst's squeamishness about the abortion issue, RU-486 is not likely to become available in the United States unless Congress becomes pro-choice enough to override a Presidential veto of the proposed Freedom of Choice Act, or a pro-choice President is elected. Another factor that might temper Hoechst's attitude toward RU-486 is the fact that German women are beginning to demand access to the drug. (Abortion was allowed in the former West Germany only up to 12 weeks and then only under very restricted conditions, but was legal and accessible on demand in the former East Germany.) There appears to be a growing political movement to make abortion more accessible in unified Germany. If abortion restrictions are eased, it might pave the way for German approval, and then, perhaps, international distribution of RU-486.

NO BLACK MARKET FOR RU-486

While RU-486 seems ensnared in Catholic politics, many advocates, including some normally staid scientists, have fantasized about cloning the drug and creating a vast underground black market. But this isn't likely to become a reality, although it is true that cloning the drug and cooking up small batches is not so difficult. China, in fact, has successfully cloned a version, and has developed its own prostaglandin as well. But manufacturing massive quantities is an expensive, multi-step process that requires pure ingredients and intensive quality control. To be effective, only precise amounts of each drug must be taken—too little or too much doesn't work, and too much may cause severe, even dangerous side effects. As for contraband supplies from Roussel stock—forget it! The company literally counts every pill. Each packet of pills leaves

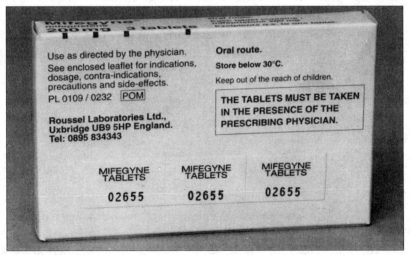

EACH PACKAGE of three RU-486 tablets is labeled with three numbered stickers. One sticker goes on factory records. The second is retained by the hospital or clinic pharmacy, and the third goes on the woman's medical chart. All labels must be accounted for at any time. With such strict controls, it is unlikely that a black market for this drug could develop.

the factory with three stickers: one for the hospital or clinic pharmacy records, one for the woman's medical records, and one to be kept by the factory—and all must be accounted for at all times. One U.S. doctor, who had wheedled a supply of the drug in a desperate attempt to save a patient who had advanced breast cancer (treatment of estrogen-dependent breast cancers is one of the many potential uses of RU-486), had to return the unused pills when the woman died.

THE ANTI-ABORTION NIGHTMARE COMES TRUE

The one bright spot on the horizon (although it will come none too soon) is that other companies, whose owners presumably don't have any problems with the abortion issue, are pursuing research into anti-progestins. Another project under research is the production of a time-release prostaglandin that will enable women to abort at home if they wish, much as they do now with normal miscarriages. In developing countries, where physicians are scarce and overworked, trained paramedics would then be able to screen out women who should not take the drug, dispense it to those who can, and counsel them on possible problems. Then the nightmares of the anti-abortion movement will have come true.

What Practitioners Need To Know About Abortion Complications

BY SHAUNA HECKERT

Executive Director, Federation of Feminist Women's Health Centers

ONE OF THE major problems in providing abortion care today is that the number of doctors who are willing to perform abortions is shrinking. Less than 30% of Ob-Gyn residency programs include specific training in abortion, and as a consequence, fewer doctors are equipped to do abortions or to treat complications when they arise.

This section reviews post-abortion complications and the recommended treatment for each. In all cases, a correct assessment of the problem allows for appropriate treatment and thus, the best possible outcome. This information is intended for practitioners who may not be familiar with abortion, but who may be called upon to do one, or who may be put in the position of treating abortion complications on an emergency basis. It may also be of interest to counselors, health educators, and others who want to learn about abortion in greater depth than in Chapter 3.

AVOIDING COMPLICATIONS

Up to 12 weeks from the last menstrual period (LMP), the risk of death or injury is exceedingly low, but these risks increase with each week of pregnancy, and are strongly influenced by the type of procedure used, whether local or general anesthesia is employed, the general health of the woman undergoing the procedure, and the skill and care of the technician performing the abortion.*

The surest way to keep abortion complications to a minimum is to:
➡ Use vacuum aspiration with a flexible plastic cannula only, avoiding the use of metal or stiff plastic instruments as much as possible.
➡ Use only a local anesthetic (or no anesthetic at all).
➡ Screen a woman carefully for preexisting conditions that might potentially cause problems and take appropriate preventive steps.
➡ Estimate gestational age as accurately as possible, using the woman's own estimation of her last normal menstrual period, and a uterine size check. If doubts exist, a Beta HCG test and a sonogram may provide helpful information. An accurate estimate of gestational age is critical in knowing which instruments to use and in judging when the abortion is complete.

---

*Most abortions are performed by physicians, but in Vermont, about 20% of abortions to 14 weeks LMP are performed by specially trained Physicians Assistants. Currently there is a movement afoot in some states to allow Nurse Practitioners to do early termination abortions as well. Therefore, I often use "practitioner" or "technician" to describe the person doing an abortion procedure.

HEALTH BACKGROUND

In the case of abortion, a complete health history isn't necessary, but taking a brief health background can be useful in eliciting the existence of some specific conditions that could complicate the procedure. **Conditions to be on the alert for include:**

➡ **Asthma:** how severe attacks are, what triggers them and what remedies are used to relieve attacks. If a woman uses an inhaler, prophylactic use shortly before the procedure may be helpful.

➡ **Epilepsy:** how often seizures occur, how severe they are, if stress or other factors are known to trigger them, and what medications, if any, she takes to control them.

➡ **Past history of pelvic inflammatory disease (PID):** Women who have had PID tend to be more susceptible to infection of the uterus, tubes, and ovaries after an abortion, and are often given antibiotics prophylactically.

➡ **Past history of tubal (ectopic) pregnancy:** Women who have had an ectopic pregnancy and still have the tube in which it occurred have a higher chance of having another pregnancy in that tube.

➡ **Fibroids:** Large fibroid growths may give the impression that the pregnancy is more advanced than it really is.

POSSIBLE BUT UNUSUAL PHYSICAL REACTIONS DURING AN ABORTION

The vast majority of abortions are completed without incident, but occasionally, unusual physical reactions can occur, and when they do, it is essential that they be handled appropriately.

➡ **Allergic reaction to local anesthesia**. Reactions to local anesthesia are rare compared to reactions and complications from general anesthesia, and are generally mild, most commonly involving a strange taste and/or ringing in the ears. Rare serious reactions may result from a toxic dose or from injecting the anesthesia directly into a blood vessel. In either case, breathing may stop suddenly and the heart can stop beating, resulting in cardiopulmonary arrest, requiring that lifesaving measures be undertaken immediately to avoid death (see "Cardiopulmonary Arrest," pages 225-226 for more detail).

➡ **Asthma attack.** Asthma, a breathing disorder caused by spasms or swelling of the bronchial tubes, usually causes no problems during an abortion, although occasionally this condition can cause a dramatic reaction, as a result of stress or a reaction to medication. At the onset of an attack, a woman may complain of having trouble breathing, and hunch forward, wheezing and gasping in an attempt to get more air.

If a woman who has asthma uses an inhaler regularly, she should bring it with her and have it at hand during the procedure. If breathing becomes difficult and the inhaler is used immediately, this will usually alleviate the condition. Reassurance and support are also helpful in lessening tension, especially in helping the woman to relax and encouraging her to control her breathing. These interventions are important, because in rare circumstances, oxygen deprivation can lead to spasms, shock, seizures, and ultimately, cardiopulmonary arrest.

➡ **Seizures.** Seizures, temporary malfunctions of the brain, can be the result of a reaction to local anesthetic, or could be one of various types of epileptic seizures, resulting from temporary changes in the normal functioning of the brain's electrical system. There are several general types of epileptic seizures: *absence seizures* (often called "petit mal"), usually lasting just a few seconds and characterized by a blank stare often followed by rapid blinking and/or chewing movements; simple *partial* *seizures* in which the person remains awake, but exhibits jerking movements in one part of the body (arm, leg or face) and may experience mental disorientation; and *generalized tonic-clonic* or "grand mal" seizures, characterized by sudden rigidity, followed by muscle jerks, shallow or temporarily suspended breathing, bluish skin and possible loss of bladder or bowel control, often followed by confusion or fatigue. Grand mal seizures can last anywhere from two to five minutes, and do not usually require further medical care unless the seizure continues for more than five minutes, or the person is injured during the seizure or is diabetic. In rare instances, grand mal seizures can result in cardiopulmonary arrest, which, if not treated immediately, can cause death. In terms of first aid, forcing an object between clenched teeth is not recommended, as it may shatter and be swallowed. A woman having a seizure should be protected from self-injury without restraining movement, her clothing loosened, and she should be turned on her side to allow her tongue to fall away from the airway and permit drainage of saliva.

➡ **Shock.** Very rarely during an abortion, shock may be caused by hemorrhage or by an allergic reaction to a drug. Signs of shock are paleness, a bluish tint to lips and nails, cool, clammy skin, dilated pupils, rapid, shallow breathing, increased heart rate but weak pulse. Women may experience mental confusion, extreme thirst, weakness, and occasionally, loss of consciousness. In the case of shock, emergency treatment is essential. The woman should be kept warm, with head lower than feet, and movement kept to a minimum until emergency help arrives. Depending on the cause, treatment may include oxygen, a blood transfusion, or injections recommended by a physician.

➡ **Cardiopulmonary arrest.** Very rarely, as a result of dilation of the cervix, allergic reactions to drugs or anesthetic, uterine perforation, or a seizure, a woman having an abortion may experience cardiac or respiratory arrest. Symptoms include pale, bluish skin, dilated pupils, no discernable heart-beat, and gasping, followed by cessation of breathing. If cardiopulmonary resuscitation (CPR) is not initiated within four to six minutes, irreversible brain damage and death can result. These events occur so rarely that medical personnel and clinic staffs may not be prepared for them. We know of one incident in a clinic that has an excellent safety record, in which a client went into cardiac arrest triggered by an asthma attack. After both the doctor and nurse had given the woman up as dead, the counselor, who was a lay health worker, revived the woman by persisting in CPR efforts. Clearly, CPR training is essential for all clinic staff, not just for medical personnel.

POST-ABORTION COMPLICATIONS

Early termination suction abortion is a very safe procedure when done by experienced practitioners under optimal conditions. According to National Abortion Federation statistics, only 3% of women under 13 weeks LMP experience complications, and only one-half of 1% require additional procedures or hospitalization. In second trimester abortions, the rate of complications increases somewhat with each succeeding week.

Nearly all abortion complications occur at the time of the abortion and will manifest themselves within the first few days after the procedure. **Possible post-abortion complications are:**
➡ retained tissue (incomplete abortion)
➡ continued pregnancy
➡ uterine infection
➡ excessive bleeding
➡ perforation of the uterus, bowel, or adjacent organs

➡ reaction to medication or anesthetic
➡ uterine tear or laceration

The three most common signs of a problem after an abortion are:
➡ pain in the abdomen or extreme cramping
➡ hemorrhage, gushing blood, large blood clots or prolonged bleeding, usually occurring only in later abortions
➡ a temperature over 100.4, sometimes accompanied by chills, which is not associated with other illness and develops within a few hours to a few days after the procedure.

If a woman is feeling well and signs of pregnancy are gone within a week (except for breast enlargement, which may take up to two weeks to subside), then it is reasonably certain that the abortion is complete. Once in a while, a missed uterine pregnancy may remain and not be detected until much later. In addition, there have been rare reports of one twin being removed (leading the practitioner to believe that the abortion is complete).

EVALUATING IF AN ABORTION IS COMPLETE

By far the most common complication of an abortion is an incomplete procedure. This problem can usually be avoided by carefully inspecting the tissue before a woman leaves the clinic. Unless she is less than three weeks pregnant, the distinctive types of tissue formation—*chorionic villi* and the *placental sac*—can be seen with the naked eye. Chorionic villi are white or yellowish, feathery cellular structures that help attach the placenta to the uterine lining. In early pregnancy, there should be a clump of villi about the size of a pencil eraser. The gestational sac is a very thin but sturdy transparent membrane that eventually develops into the "bag of waters" as the pregnancy nears term. Two distinguishing characteristics of the sac are that it is difficult to tear, and it floats when immersed in water.

After the abortion, the uterine contents should be carefully examined for chorionic villi and the placental sac. Unless the pregnancy is extremely early, before four weeks LMP, both must be present to ensure that the abortion is complete. Fetal parts are rarely seen before nine to 10 weeks LMP. If no tissue is obtained during the procedure, there are three possibilities: 1) the pregnancy has been missed, or 2) the pregnancy is in the egg tube (an ectopic pregnancy—see pages 238-239), or 3) the woman had a false positive pregnancy test and was not pregnant to begin with. (False positive blood pregnancy tests are rare, but can be caused by certain tranquilizers, barbiturates, marijuana, methadone, psychotropic drugs, anti-depressants, and anti-convulsants.)

INCOMPLETE ABORTION

If, after the abortion, some tissue or large blood clots have not been removed, the uterus will contract in an effort to expel the remaining tissue or clots, and a woman will experience heavy cramping. Left alone, the uterus will sometimes expel the retained tissue, but the chances that it won't are too high count on. **If an incomplete abortion is suspected, the most important thing that should be done is a second aspiration (often called *reaspiration*).** If a re-aspiration appears warranted, there are two compelling reasons for doing it as soon as possible:

➡ the longer the tissue is left in the uterus, the greater the chance of infections;

➡ the woman will feel better quickly when her abortion is complete.

Twenty years of experience with legal abortion has revealed that even tiny amounts of retained tissue can cause heavy cramping. Doctors who are not experienced with abortion may not be aware of the necessity of reaspiration and may choose to treat a woman inappropriately with antibiotics.

THE BENEFITS OF REASPIRATION OR D&C

In the past, women with incomplete abortions or impending miscarriages were given antibiotics for several days before a respiration or D&C was done. This outdated practice was based on the rationale that an infection had developed, and that a second procedure might spread it or make it worse. However, if there is retained tissue in the uterus causing an infection, antibiotics will not clear up the infection until the tissue is removed. In this case delay may increase the possibility of bleeding, hemorrhage, or infection. Fever resulting from retained tissue subsides after the reaspiration.

In the case of a suspected incomplete abortion, the well-established guideline recommended by the Centers for Disease Control is: **When in doubt, reaspirate.**

CONTINUED PREGNANCY

Within one week after an abortion, all signs of pregnancy should have vanished, and by two to three weeks after the procedure, a pregnancy test should be negative. If it has been two weeks since the procedure and a woman still feels pregnant, there is a good chance that she still is. Sometimes, however, a woman does not realize that she is pregnant until much later, due to stress or an underlying illness with similar symptoms, and if it is too late to do an abortion, she and her practitioner may worry that the

fetus has been damaged. Often, however, if the fetus continues to grow, it has probably not been affected by the
attempted abortion.

Pregnancy tests may be helpful in evaluating a continued pregnancy, but in this case, a uterine size check is
the most reliable marker. Approximately one to three
women in 1,000 will have a continued (or missed) pregnancy, in which the fetus remains intact and continues to
grow. On rare occasions, women have remained pregnant,
even though chorionic villi was seen at the time of the procedure.

UNANTICIPATED LATER ABORTION

Hemorrhage, or heavy bleeding during or in the days following an early termination suction abortion, is exceedingly rare. When it does occur, it is usually because the
pregnancy has advanced beyond 12 weeks and is larger
than was initially estimated. In later abortions, if the pregnancy has been interrupted but fetal parts are trapped
inside the uterus, hemorrhage can occur during the procedure, creating a serious situation. In this case, the abortion should be completed that day by a skilled surgeon in
a hospital.

Another unexpected complication of later abortion
that can occur is tearing or laceration of the uterus or cervical canal, which result in hemorrhage or a steady ooze of
blood. A skilled technician may be able to stitch the site of
the tear and control the bleeding.

DILATION AND EVACUATION

Until the late 1970s, late abortions, if they were done at
all, were done by saline induction or *hysterotomy*, a sort of
early cesarean procedure. Some doctors who did abortions
were always pushing the limits, often because of the diffi-

culties in estimating gestational age, but at other times because they were too kind-hearted to turn a desperate woman away, even though they might suspect that she was past what was normally considered safe. Finding themselves in such situations, doctors often improvised, inserting more laminaria, perhaps on successive days (see page 90), using larger cannulas, and using forceps to remove fetal parts. What they found, much to their surprise, was that the procedure they developed, called dilation and evacuation, or D&E was much safer, took far less time staff time, and was psychologically far less traumatic for the woman, than saline abortions or hysterotomies.

DIFFERENCES BETWEEN EARLY TERMINATION SUCTION ABORTION AND D&E

There are many similarities between early termination suction procedures and D&E abortions, but there are also some striking differences.

➡ Early suction abortion can be done in one visit, with an optional follow-up visit if needed or desired, whereas a D&E requires three or sometimes four visits, one or two to have laminaria inserted, one for the procedure (which may or may not be done on the day of the laminaria insertion), and a follow-up visit.

➡ After 18 weeks, D&Es usually require general anesthesia.

➡ After 20 weeks, many clinics give an injection of *digoxin immune fab (Ovine)* (Digibind), normally used as an antidote for severe digitalis toxicity or overdose. A small dose of digoxin stops the fetal heartbeat *in utero* making the removal of fetal parts easier.

➡ Because of complex factors that cause a woman to seek a later abortion, a D&E is often a more difficult experience for her. Factors that cause women to delay getting an abortion are denial, a genuine failure to recognize the signs of pregnancy, ambivalence about continuing the pregnancy, difficulty in getting money, lack of access to abortion services, and parental notification requirements.

ABNORMAL BLEEDING

Spotting or light to period-like bleeding is normal after an abortion. A woman may even pass a few dime- to quarter-sized blood clots in the first 12 to 24 hours, especially if she normally has them during her period.

Abnormal heavy bleeding or hemorrhage is usually defined as bleeding through a standard-sized menstrual pad in less than an hour, continuing for several hours. Another abnormal bleeding pattern is a "gush" of blood, which may occur several times with no bleeding in between. Blood clots that are very large, i.e., about the size of the palm of your hand, are also considered to be abnormal.

These abnormal bleeding patterns most commonly occur because of an incomplete abortion. Normally, uterine contractions, which control bleeding, do not occur as readily when there is retained tissue. Instead, the uterus attempts to flush the tissue out by increased bleeding. Sometimes this works: Women pass the retained tissue themselves, and bleeding subsides to expected levels. If the bleeding does not decrease, however, a reaspiration is usually done to avoid the possibility of an incomplete abortion.

Another possible, but less likely, cause of heavy bleeding is the failure of the uterus to contract to its prepregnant size because it lacks adequate tone or strength, due to ill health (especially I.V. drug use), poor nutrition, or multiple childbirths.

A steady ooze of blood coming from the vagina shortly after abortion could be from poor uterine muscle tone, but it could also be a sign that a perforation has occurred. (See "Perforation" page 235).

CONTROL OF ABNORMAL BLEEDING

Methergine (methylergonovine maleate) is a prescription drug derived from ergot, an herb that causes uterine contractions and is commonly used after abortion, miscarriage, and birth to cause the uterus to contract to help control bleeding. Methergine is not particularly useful in expelling retained tissue, but it can be very helpful in contracting the uterus, especially if a woman's uterus is weak or has poor muscle tone. If bleeding does not subside to an acceptable level after giving methergine, the best solution is probably reaspiration.

Uterine massage. If cramping is due to retained blood clots, massaging the uterus by firmly pressing across the abdomen towards the pubic mound may help expel them. Uterine massage, however, is unlikely to expel retained tissue. If cramps persist after one to two hours, a reaspiration is probably necessary.

Ice packs. Ice packs placed on the abdomen for 15 or 20 minutes can help constrict blood vessels and bring bleeding under control. Heat, which will increase bleeding, is contraindicated, even though the woman may be having severe cramps. If the bleeding is due to an incomplete abortion, ice packs won't help.

DISSEMINATED INTRAVASCULAR COAGULATION (DIC)

Prolonged oozing of blood or hemorrhage (heavy blood loss over a few hours) may lead to a rare syndrome usually associated with late second trimester abortions, called *disseminated intravascular coagulation* (DIC). After a certain critical amount of blood has been lost, the blood is depleted of *fibrinogen* and loses its ability to clot, appearing thin and watery. In advanced DIC, if a woman recently had blood drawn from a finger poke or from her arm, she may begin bleeding from these sites as well. **DIC is a serious, life-threatening condition that will not resolve on its own, and can only be reversed by an immediate blood transfusion,** which should bring the fibrinogen back up to an acceptable level within 24 hours.

PROLONGED BLEEDING

Bleeding three to four weeks post-abortion is somewhat abnormal, and may signify an incomplete procedure; a reaspiration may reveal some retained tissue. Occasionally, however, spotting occurs, steadily or off and on, until a woman gets her period again (typically in four to eight weeks), and may or may not indicate retained tissue. If tissue is retained, it is sometimes expelled during the first normal period. Other times, a reaspiration may be necessary.

SEVERE CRAMPING WITHOUT BLEEDING ("POST-ABORTION SYNDROME")

Occasionally, a woman's cervix closes, as if in spasm, and won't allow blood to flow out freely. The uterus can fill with blood and clots, distending to the size of a 10 to 12 week pregnant uterus, and become very tender to the touch. In this case, reaspiration will open the cervical canal and remove the blood and clots. Women usually feel better immediately, and rarely need further treatment.

TEMPERATURE OVER 100.4°F

Women can run a low-grade fever for many reasons, but if the temperature is elevated to 100.4 shortly after an abortion, this is usually a sign of a uterine infection, indicating that there is retained tissue. In this case, the uterus will feel tender, especially during a bi-manual exam. If there is retained tissue, the infection will not clear up, even if antibiotics are administered, until the retained tissue is expelled by the uterus itself or until it is removed by reaspiration. Afterward, if a woman is in good health, the infection may resolve on its own, but antibiotics may be necessary to completely eradicate it.

Occasionally, post-abortion fever may be caused by other factors such as flu or a severe urinary tract infection. If a woman's general health is poor, if she has a history of pelvic inflammatory disease, or other pre-existing infection such as gonorrhea, her temperature may rise. In these cases, antibiotics are recommended.

THE CONSEQUENCES OF AN UNTREATED UTERINE INFECTION

When abortion was illegal in the United States, infections as a result of incomplete abortion, or *sepsis*, resulted in the deaths of many women. Legalization, however, virtually eradicated this condition. Left untreated, the infection gradually spreads to the blood stream and vital organs (perhaps in conjunction with a perforation of the uterus or bowel), creating a life-threatening situation.

A uterine infection that is unrelated to an incomplete abortion will most likely linger, frequently spreading to the egg tubes and ovaries and becoming full-blown pelvic inflammatory disease (PID). Symptoms of PID are general pain in the abdomen, or a sharp pain on one side or the other. Over time, the infection can cause abscesses and scarring of the egg tubes and can result in infertility.

PERFORATION

Perforation, a tear or puncture of the uterine wall, occurred fairly frequently when many abortions were done by untrained practitioners who used curettes and other sharp metal instruments, or when women attempted to induce their own miscarriages with coat hangers, knitting needles, wires, and other instruments. With the advent of flexible plastic cannulas and suction equipment, serious perforations requiring clinical attention have become one of the least likely complications. Nonetheless, any time instruments such as curettes, dilators, and in later abortion, forceps, are introduced into the uterus, the potential for perforation is greater. Ideally, only a flexible cannula is used.

Rushing to complete an abortion is one factor that increases the risk of perforation. The safest abortions are not hurried, and the practitioner performing the procedure is assisted by experienced staff who work well together as a team. Communication during the procedure between the woman and staff, which is possible if local anesthesia is employed, is a factor that helps reduce the risk of perforation. In addition, a woman who is awake can report any pain that might indicate that dilators or the cannula is being inserted too far or too forcefully into the uterus.

In some cases, when a small uterus is perforated with a small cannula, a perforation goes unnoticed by both the woman and the practitioner, and the uterus heals on its own. This phenomenon has occasionally been observed when a perforation occurs during a routine uterine evacuation preceding a tubal ligation. The site of the perforation is later discovered by the doctor using a laparoscope at the time of the sterilization procedure.

In other instances, the practitioner may feel an instrument "give" as it pierces the uterine wall and enters the abdominal cavity. The woman may feel a sharp pain, especially with a cough or sudden movement. She may also feel faint and her bleeding can be heavy. If the practitioner suspects a perforation, it is best to stop and monitor the woman's reaction. Simple perforations, i.e, those that pierce only the uterine wall, are generally not serious, but those that also include perforation of the bowel, bladder, or uterine artery can be life-threatening.

UNCOMPLICATED UTERINE PERFORATIONS

If the perforation occurs at the completion of the abortion, if all of the tissue has been removed, and no other organs are damaged, the uterus will most likely heal on its own. If the woman is not in pain and has no fever or hemorrhage, she will probably need no further medical attention. In this case, many practitioners give oxytocin and a course of antibiotics, but this is more of a precaution than a necessity. Oxytocin is a pituitary hormone that, among other actions, causes the uterus to contract during labor. Pitocin, a synthetic analog of oxytocin, is used to increase contractions and speed labor, and is also sometimes used to cause the uterus to contract after an abortion.

If the perforation occurs before tissue has been obtained, the clinical picture is similar to that described above. Most clinicians stop the procedure and wait a week or two for the uterus to heal before proceeding, prescribing antibiotics as a precaution.

SERIOUS, COMPLICATED PERFORATIONS

If the perforation happens in the middle of the abortion, after some but not all of the tissue has been removed, there is the potential for infection and hemorrhage just as there is for incomplete abortion (see page 228).

In this case, there are two specific options for completing the abortion safely:
➡ if an ultrasound machine is available, and the clinician is very experienced, he or she may attempt to complete the procedure, using the ultrasound as a guide to avoid reentering the perforation.

➡ if laparoscopic equipment is available on site or at a nearby hospital, the clinician may attempt to complete the abortion while monitoring the perforation area with a laparoscope.

If the perforation goes through the uterus and punctures the bowel additional surgical measures must be undertaken to repair the bowel, generally involving removing the damaged portion. If a significant portion of the bowel is removed, the woman may need a temporary or permanent colostomy. This drastic procedure was much more common in the days of illegal abortion when metal instruments were routinely employed in terminating pregnancies.

If the perforation involves the uterine artery, heavy bleeding may result, and if left untreated, could lead to shock and ultimately, cardiopulmonary arrest. Unfortunately, artery involvement is not always evident at the time of perforation. If the woman is still in the clinic, the standard practice is to monitor pain and look for signs of internal bleeding for a couple of hours. In rare instances where a uterine artery has been damaged, hysterectomy (removal of uterus, but not the ovaries) may be the only remedy.

ECTOPIC PREGNANCY

If a woman has a positive pregnancy test, but no tissue is obtained during the abortion, this may be a sign of an ectopic (tubal) pregnancy. Sometimes these errant pregnancies, which are most commonly found in the egg tubes, simply fail to thrive and calcify or are reabsorbed. Usually, however, an ectopic pregnancy continues to grow, and if it is not removed surgically, at between eight and 10 weeks gestation, it will rupture the egg tube, precipitating a life-threatening situation. Women who have a history of PID or previous ectopic pregnancies are at highest risk for this condition.

Early signs of an unruptured ectopic pregnancy—vague abdominal pain and tenderness, usually on one side, and sometimes bleeding or spotting—may be deceiving or may not be taken seriously. Signs of an impending rupture are more dramatic, including severe abdominal pain, dizziness and fainting, pallor, and possibly shock. The definitive way to diagnose an ectopic pregnancy is by ultrasound or laparoscopy. After pinpointing the site of the pregnancy, it must be removed surgically, and the tube may or may not be saved, depending on the skill of the surgeon and how advanced the pregnancy is.

THE IMPORTANCE OF FOLLOW-UP

Post-abortion complications usually show up within the first week after the procedure, but occasionally a woman may not notice signs of an incomplete abortion until the second week or rarely, even later. Women should be given clear information about potential problems and be made to feel comfortable about reporting a problem. If a woman does not have confidence in her provider, she may panic if she experiences pain or heavy bleeding, and may seek the help of other practitioners, who may not be equipped to deal with the problem appropriately.

The Del-Em™

LORRAINE ROTHMAN, the inventor of the Del-EM™ applied for and received a patent in 1974, and notes that she did so to document the fact that it had been developed by a women's health activist. At our request, Lorraine described Del-Em™ assembly in order to demystify its manufacture. She retains the exclusive right to distribute the Del-Em™ commercially.

SUPPLIES (see Resource List for suppliers, page 248).
Canning jar (1/2 pint; alternative: any jar or glass the rubber stopper will fit tightly)
Rubber stopper (#13 two-hole, chemistry lab variety)
Medical or aquarium tubing (15" and 30" segments; clear tubing is ideal, but rubber catheter tubing is also acceptable)
Cannulas (4mm, 5mm, 6mm)
60cc syringe (disposable plastic)
Automatic two-way bypass valve
5mm cannula (to be cut for valve adaptor and adaptor for 4mm cannula)
6mm cannula (to be cut for adaptors for rubber stoppers)
Water soluble lubricating jelly
Toothpicks or coffee stirring sticks
Knife or single-edged razor blade
Cutting board

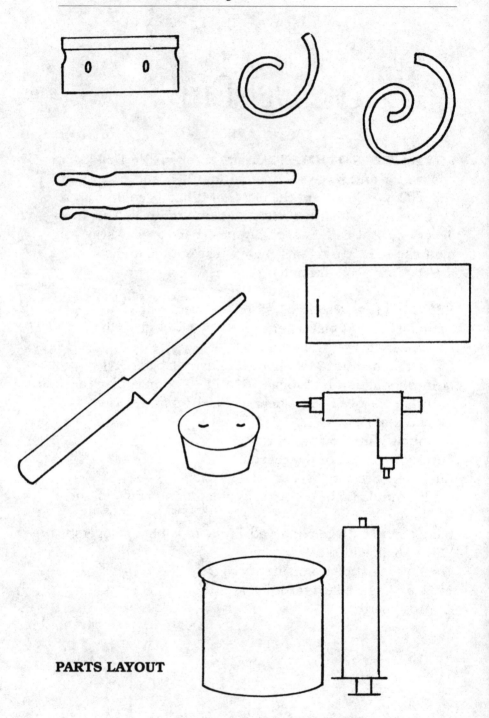

PARTS LAYOUT

ASSEMBLY

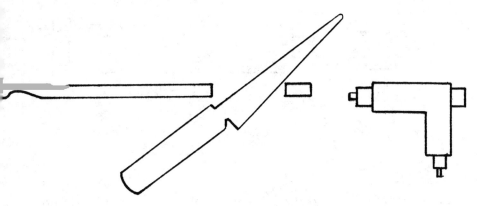

1. Hold the 5mm cannula flat on the cutting board and cut two 1" pieces. Save one piece for use later. Attach the other piece to the valve by holding the adaptor firmly between the fingers of one hand and the valve between the fingers in the other hand, pushing until the adaptor is completely over the valve post and feels tight and unmovable.

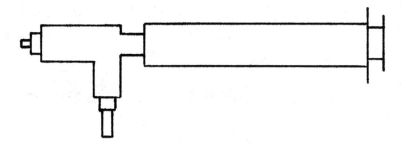

2. Attaching the valve to the syringe: The Leur-lok valve requires a Leur-lok syringe and has a screw-on connection. Other valves can be attached to the syringe by pressing firmly.

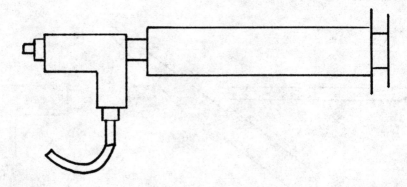

3. Attach the shorter (15") piece of tubing to the adaptor on the valve, hold the tube firmly in one hand and the adaptor end of the valve with the other hand. Press the tubing firmly to the valve, pushing it on as far as it will.

4. To make adaptor insertion easier, moisten the holes in the stopper with a water soluble lubricant, coaxing lubricant into the holes with a stiffener such as toothpicks or a coffee stirring stick.

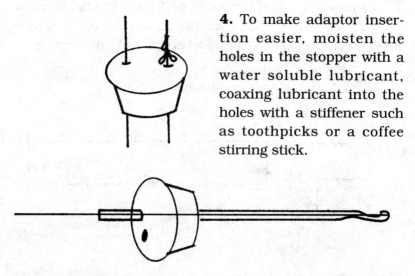

5. Hold the 6mm cannula firmly and force the rounded end into the lubricated hole at the top of the rubber stopper. If the cannula does not push through easily, insert stiffener into it to make it firmer and force the cannula through until 1" is left coming out of the top of the hole it first entered.

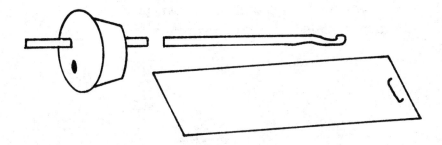

6. With one hand, hold the rubber stopper with the cannula lying against the cutting board, and with the other hand cut the 6mm cannula so that the 1/2" of the tube is left protruding from the bottom of the rubber stopper.

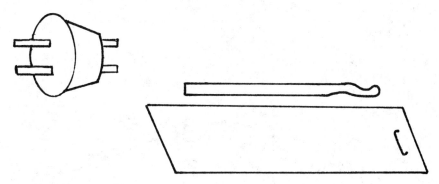

7. Follow the same steps as in 5. and 6. above to put tube into second stopper hole.

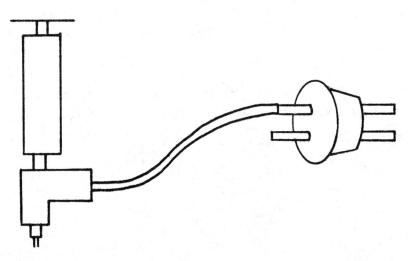

8. Attach the other end of the shorter (15") tube to a 1" tube on the top of the rubber stopper, pressing firmly to get a tight fit, like this:

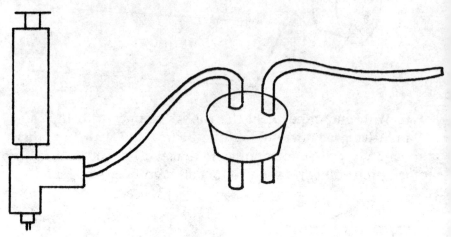

9. Attach the longer piece of tubing (30") to the second tube on the top of the rubber stopper, pressing firmly, like this:

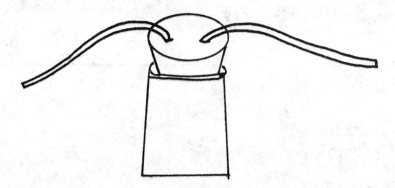

10. Holding the glass jar firmly with one hand, press the bottom of the rubber stopper into the jar opening, making sure that the rubber stopper fits tightly, like this:

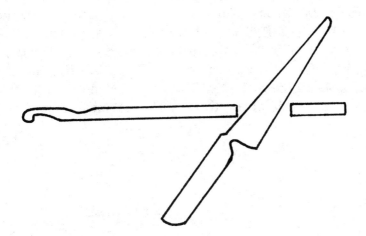

11. If a 4mm cannula is to be used, prepare the adaptor so that the cannula will fit firmly on the tubing by cutting a one" piece of the 5mm cannula.

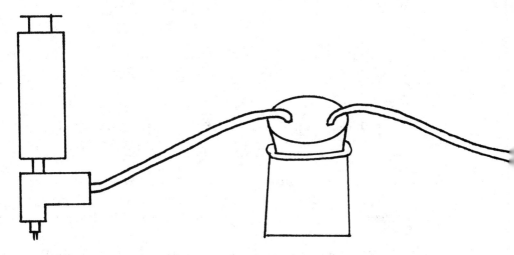

12. Attach the 1" adaptor to the end of the 30" piece of tubing by pressing firmly.

Note: When a 5mm or 6mm cannula is occasionally used in menstrual extraction, the 1" adaptor for the tubing is not needed.

13. Attach the cannula by holding the open end firmly between the fingers of one hand. In the other hand, hold the end of the 30" piece of tubing, which will also have the 1" adaptor (if a 4mm cannula is being used). Press the cannula end into the tubing very firmly so that the cannula is being held tightly. The cannula end should be at least 1/2" inside of the tubing. The finished kit looks like this:

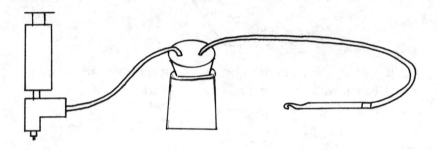

POSSIBLE SOURCES OF SUPPLY FOR DEL-EM™ PARTS & ACCESSORIES

JARS: Pint-size canning jars, standard size opening of the type obtained from most large supermarkets and grocery stores that stock canning and jelly-making equipment.

TUBING: TygonR formulation R-3603 (or similar quality), inside diameter 3/16", outside diameter 5/16", wall 1/16", are often obtained from teachers' and students' laboratory and science stores in local communities. These are listed in Business Yellow Pages under "Laboratory and Scientific Supplies." Items not kept in stock may be listed in a supplier's catalog, or special ordered. Comparable tubing is sometimes obtained at hardware and tropical fish stores.

A. DIAGGER AND CO., (800) 321-8937, Richmond CA, mail-order catalog catering to public school science teachers and students.

NEBRASKA SCIENTIFIC, (800) 228-7117. Catalog #S73651-C. Will ship pre-paid orders to individuals.

SARGENT WELCH LABORATORY SUPPLIES, (800). Supply tubing in lengths of 10, 50 and 100 feet.

SCIENTIFIC PRODUCTS, A DIVISION OF BAXTER HEALTHCARE CORP., (800) 553-2913, (800) 553-2913, sells only to companies with established accounts. 10 ft. (T6020-2), 50 ft. (T-010-2), and 100 ft. (T-01000-2T).

VAN WATERS AND ROGERS (800) 999-4VWR, sells only to companies with established accounts.

RUBBER STOPPERS, NO. 13, TWO HOLE: Generally obtained from above suppliers.

SYRINGES:60 cc. B and D (Becton Dickinson) plastic polypropylene. Available from Nebraska Scientific, Sargent Welch, Scientific Products, and Van Waters and Rogers.

AUTOMATIC TWO-WAY PLASTIC VALVE:

LUX SCIENTIFIC INSTRUMENT CORP. (602) 327-4848, Dual check valve No. 91-057-070. Catalog, sells to prepaid company accounts.

B-D (BECTON DICKINSON) AND CORNWALL PIPETTER stainless steel valves, equivalent to Dual check valve. May be available through above suppliers.

CANNULAS: These distributors sell cannulas in small quantities to businesses only.

Manufacturers

BERKELEY MEDEVICES
907 Camelia St.
Berkeley CA 94710
(510) 526-4046 (in CA only)
(800) 227-2388

LABORATORIES LUNEAU
B.P. 252-28005
Chartres, France
387 25 25

Distributors: These distributors sell cannulas to businesses only.

ACCORD
3775 Via Nona Marie, #210
Carmel CA 93923
(800) 556-2255

BERKELEY MEDEVICES
907 Camelia St.
Berkeley CA 94710
(510) 526-4046 (in CA only)
(800) 227-2388

CABOT MEDICAL
2021 Cabott Blvd., W.
Langhorne, PA 19047

INTERNATIONAL PROJECTS ASSISTANCE
SERVICE (IPAS)
P.O. Box 100
Carrboro, NC 27510
(800) 334-8446

MED GYN PRODUCTS, INC.
2808 A Center Circle Dr.
Downers Grove, IL 60515
(800) 451-9667

When cannulas are not available, women have sometimes purchased 4mm tubing in bulk and fashion it into cannulas using an Exacto knife or single-edged razor blade and sealing one end with a heat source, such as an iron or light bulb.

References

WHY THIS BOOK IS NECESSARY, pp. 1–6.

1. S. K. Henshaw & J. Van Vort, "Abortion Services in the United States, 1878 and 1988," *Family Planning Perspectives* 22:102, 1990.

2. R.B. Gold, *Abortion and Women's Health*, The Alan Guttmacher Institute, 1990, p. 27.

3. Gallup Organization poll, June, 1992. The question was, "Do you think abortions should be legal under all circumstances, only certain circumstances, or illegal in all circumstances?" Cited in "Public Support for Abortion," National Abortion Federation Fact Sheet, August 1990.

4. ABC Poll, 1990. Cited in "Public Support for Abortion," National Abortion Federation Fact Sheet, August 1990.

CHAPTER 1. FINDING AN ABORTION PROVIDER, pp. 7–48.

1. "The Economics of Abortion," National Abortion Federation Fact Sheet, January, 1991.

2. Ibid.

3. Women's Health Education Project, *Abortion: A New York City Resource Guide*, 1992, p. 65-66.

4. Testimony of Dr. Edward Ehlinger in the case of *Hodgson v. Minnesota* Civ. No. 3-81538 (D. Minn. January 23, 1985), cited in *Parental Notice Laws: Their Catastrophic Impact on Teenagers' Right to Abortion*, The Reproductive Freedom Project of the American Civil Liberties Union, 1986, p. 7.

5. A. Torres, J.D. Forrest & S. Eisman, "Telling Parents: Clinic Policies and Adolescents' Use of Family Planning and Abortion Services," *Family Planning Perspectives* (12) 1980, pp. 284.

6. *Ibid.*, p. 288.

7. The Reproductive Freedom Project of the American Civil Liberties Union Foundation, *No Way Out: Young, Pregnant and Trapped by the Law*, 1991, p. 6.

8. Torres, p. 287.

9. Bill Bell, "Dear Becky: Letter to All Daughters from a Father," *Seventeen*, March, 1991, p. 184.

10. Sue Halpern, "Teen-Abortion Law Turns Trauma into Tragedy," *Rolling Stone*, Aug. 9, 1990, p. 43.

11. American Civil Liberties Association Reproductive Freedom Project, *Parental Notice Laws: Their Catastrophic Impact on Teenagers' Right to Abortion*, 1986, p. 12.

12. Ibid., p. 13.

13. Op. cit., WHEP, p. 64-65.

14. J. Belsky, "Medically Indigent Women Seeking Abortion Prior to Legalization: New York City, 1969-1970," *Family Planning Perspectives*, 24, 1992.

15. L.C. Phelan and P.T. Maginnis, *The Abortion Handbook* (North Hollywood, CA; Contact Books, 1969), pp. 111-115.

16. D.F. Papolos, M.D., and J. Papolos, *Overcoming Depression* (New York; Harper Collins, 1987), p. 3.

17. R.M. Soderstrom, "A Manual Vacuum Syringe for Uterine Evacuation," *Contemporary OB/GYN*, April 15, 1991, pp. 2-3.

18. Op. cit. Phelan, p. 151.

CHAPTER 3, THE BEST AVAILABLE ABORTION CARE, pp. 67–96

1. National Abortion Federation Fact Sheet, "Safety of Abortion," April 1992.

2. R.B. Gold, *Abortion and Women's Health: A Turning Point for America*, The Alan Guttmacher Institute, 1990, p. 29.

3. C.E. Koop, Letter to President Ronald Reagan, January 9, 1989.

4. Op. cit. Gold, p. 35.

5. B. Ehrenreich, *New York Times*, Feb. 7, 1985.

CHAPTER 4, BACK TO THE BAD OLD DAYS? pp. 97–111.

1. S. Barr, *A Woman's Choice*, (New York: Rawson Associates, 1977), out of print.

2. R. Barnett, as told to D. Baker, *They Weep on My Doorstep* Beaverton, OR; Halo Publishers, 1969, p. 74. (See Suggested Reading, p. TK, for ordering information.)

3. L.C. Phelan and P.T. Maginnis, *The Abortion Handbook* (North Hollywood, CA; Contact Books, 1969).

CHAPTER 5, THE DEVELOPMENT OF MENSTRUAL EXTRACTION, pp. 112–128.

1. R. Amin, et al., "Menstrual Regulation Training and Service Programs in Bangladesh: Results from a National Survey," *Studies in Family Planning*, 20:2, 1989, p. 102-106.

2. E. Royston and S. Armstrong, *Preventing Maternal Deaths*, World Health Organization, 1989, and L. Liskin, "Complications of Abortion in Developing Countries," *Population Reports*, Series F, No. 7, 1980.

3. F.A. Moeloek, et al., "The Relation Between Menstrual Regulation service and the Incidence of Septic Abortions in Indonesia," p. 2. Available from International Women's Health Coalition, 24 East 21st Street, New York, NY 10010.

CHAPTER 8, THE LEGALITY OF MENSTRUAL EXTRACTION, pp. 167–182.

1. C. Smith-Rosenberg, *Disorderly Conduct: Visions of Gender in Victorian America*, (New York: Knopf, 1985), p. 220.

2. "Brief of 250 American Historians as Amici Curiae in Support of Planned Parenthood of Southeastern Pennsylvania, in *Planned Parenthood of Southeastern Pennsylvania, et al., v. Robert P. Casey, et al.*, in the Supreme Court of the United States, October Term, 1991," p. 1.

3. Smith-Rosenberg, pp. 217-244.

4. J. Mohr, *Abortion in America: The Origins and Evolution of National Policy* (New York and Oxford: Oxford University Press, 1978).

5. L. Lader, *Abortion* (New York: Bobbs-Merrill Co., 1966).

6. R. P. Petchesky, *Abortion and Woman's Choice: The State, Sexuality, and Reproductive Freedom,* (Boston: Northeastern University Press, 1984), pp. 67-100.

7. K. Luker, *Abortion and the Politics of Motherhood,* (Berkeley: University of California Press, 1984), pp. 11-39.

8. B. Ehrenrich and D. English, *For Her Own Good: 150 Years of the Experts' Advice to Women,* (New York; Anchor Press/Doubleday, 1979), p. 51.

9. The Boston Women's Health Book Collective, *The New Our Bodies, Ourselves,* (New York: Simon & Schuster, revised edition in press).

CHAPTER 9, HERBS AND OTHER TRADITIONAL METHODS OF FERTILITY CONTROL, pp. 183–202.

1. J.M. Riddle, *Contraception and Abortion from the Ancient World to the Renaissance* (Cambridge: Harvard University Press, 1992.)

2. *Wise Woman Herbal* (Woodstock, NY; Ash Tree Press, 1986). Susan Weed mentions two isolated reports of groups of women, one in Northern California and one in a village in India, who reportedly used wild carrot seeds successfully for pregnancy prevention, but there is no way to verify either of these reports.

3. J.B. Sullivan, et al, "Pennyroyal Oil Poisoning and Hepatotoxicity," *Journal of the American Medical Association,* 242:2873, 1979.

4. E.P. Samborskaia, "The Mechanism of Artificial Abortion by Use of Ascorbic Acid," *Biulleten Eksperimental'noi Biologii i Meditsiny,* Vol 62, pp. 96-98 1966. Cited in Irwin Stone, *The Healing Factor: Vitamin C Against Disease* (New York; Grosset & Dunlap, 1977).

5. *Physician's Desk Reference* (Oradell, N.J.; Medical Economics Company, Inc., 1992, 46th ed.) p. 2159.

6. P.S. Schonhofer, "Brazil: Misuse of Misoprostol as an Abortifacient May Induce Malformations," *The Lancet,* (337) 1534-1535, 1991.

7. Op. cit., Schonhofer.

CHAPTER 10, FOLK METHODS THAT ARE DANGEROUS AND DON'T WORK, pp. 203–206.

1. Op. cit., Phelan and Maginnis, p. 135.

CHAPTER 11, IS RU-486 THE WAVE OF THE FUTURE? pp. 207–220

1. L.K. Altman, "A Simpler Way to Employ Ru-486 Is Reported," *New York Times*, April 9, 1991.

2. "Contragestion and Other Clinical Applications of RU-486, an Antiprogesterone at the Receptor," E.-E. Baulieu, *Science*, Sept. 22, 1989, p. 1355.

3. Personal interview with Rev. Ken Dupin, RCR Alliance (now defunct) by Rebecca Chalker, April 27, 1990.

4. S. Greenhouse, "A Fierce Battle: Politics and profits: The French abortion pill RU-486 sparked bitter controversy but finally survived," *New York Times Magazine*, Feb. 12, 1989, p. 24.

5. W. Koberstein, "Edouard Sakiz: From Paris with "Art—Roussel-Uclaf Paints a Global Future," *Pharmaceutical Executive*, January, 1990, p. 30.

Suggested Reading

ABORTION

ABORTION, Lawrence Lader (Indianapolis: Bobbs-Merrill, 1966). This early study documents laws and practices governing abortion in the United States and around the world, and makes a powerful case for abortion reform.

ABORTION II: MAKING THE REVOLUTION, Lawrence Lader (New York: Beacon Press, 1973). In this sequel to Abortion, Lader chronicles the history of the abortion reform movement, with information on strtegy, the feminist role, clergy referral services, and important leaders.

ABORTION: THE CLASH OF ABSOLUTES, Laurence H. Tribe (New York: W.W. Norton & Co., 1990). Written by a well-known Harvard law professor, this illuminating book takes a look at abortion from a philosophical/legal perspective.

THE ABORTION FACTBOOK, 1992, Stanley K. Henshaw and Jennifer van Vort (New York: Allan Guttmacher Institute, 1992). This is Guttmacher's annual report on abortion, with statistics and analyses on virtually every facet of the abortion issue.

ABORTION WITHOUT APOLOGY: A RADICAL HISTORY FOR THE 1990S, Ninia Baehr (Boston: South End Press, Pamphlet No. 8, 1990). A concise history of the struggle for abortion and reproductive rights in the United States, clearly delineating the distinctions between the "radical" perspective, which calls for repeal of all laws on abortion, and the "reformist" perspective, which advocates physician-only abortions and the 24-week limit for abortions.

ABORTION AND WOMEN'S CHOICE: THE STATE, SEXUALITY, AND REPRODUCTIVE FREEDOM, by Rosalind Pollack Petchesky (Boston: Northeastern University Press, 1984). An exhaustively researched and cogently argued study of the impact of abortion laws on society, sexuality, and women's lives.

BACK ROOMS: AN ORAL HISTORY OF THE ILLEGAL ABORTION MOVEMENT, Ellen Messer and Kathryn E. May (New York: Simon & Schuster, 1988). Chilling, compelling memoirs of women and men, doctors and activists, who remember life, sex, and abortion before *Roe v. Wade*.

259

CREATING COMMON GROUND: WOMEN'S PERSPECTIVES ON THE SELECTION AND INTRODUCTION OF FERTILITY REGULATION TECHNOLOGIES, World Health Organization Special Program of Research, Development and Research Training in Human Reproduction (Geneva) and International Women's Health Coalition (24 E. 21st. St., New York, NY 10010), 1991. This document summarizes the results of a meeting between women's health advocates and scientists which explored differences in approaches to fertility regualtion and contraceptive research, and proposes that these two groups work together to enhance the appropriateness and acceptability of developing contraceptive technologies.

FACING A FUTURE WITHOUT CHOICE: A REPORT ON REPRODUCTIVE LIBERTY IN AMERICA, National Abortion Rights Action League (NARAL) and the NARAL Foundation, (1101 14th St., N.W., Wahingtion, DC 20005), 1992. This report summarizes the findings of a commission of experts assembled by NARAL to evaluate the consequences of losing the freedom to choose, and to recommend strategies to safeguard reproductive freedom.

FROM ABORTION TO REPRODUCTIVE FREEDOM: TRANSFORMING A MOVEMENT, Marlene Gerber Fried (Boston: South End Press, 1990). This anthology, unprecedented in its cultural diversity, brings together activists, journalists, and academics, all deeply involved in fighting for women's health and political power. They present a history and critique of the aboriton rights struggle from the late 1960s to the present and argue for an expansion of the single-issue abortion-rights movement into a multi-cultural feminist movement.

HAVING AN ABORTION? YOUR GUIDE TO GOOD CARE/?VA A HACERSE UN ABORTO? GUIA PARA OBTENER BUENA ATENCION, Ann Thompson Cook, translated by Stephanie Siefken (1990) single copies $.75. Available from the National Abortion Federation, 1434 U St., N.W., Washington, D.C. 20009, (800) 772-9100.

LIFE ITSELF: ABORTION IN THE AMERICAN MIND, Roger Rosenblatt (New York: Random House, 1992). Written by a journalist and social commentator, this book traces the history of social thought about abortion and examines American attitudes toward life in general, and abortion in particular.

THE NEW OUR BODIES, OURSELVES, Boston Women's Health Book Collective (New York: Simon & Schuster, 1984; updated edition due in late 1992). This classic, authoritiative women's health resource encompasses abortion, reproductive health and childbearing, as well as a variety of social and lifestyle issues.

A NEW VIEW OF A WOMAN'S BODY, The Federation of Feminist Women's Health Centers, 1080 N. Vine St., #1105, Los Angeles, CA 90028, ($19.95 + $2.50 p/h). Suzann Gage's beautiful, informative illustrations provide an eye-opening look at women's sexual and reproductive anatomy and physiology. This book includes landmark chapters on menstrual extraction and women's sexual anatomy.

REPRODUCTIVE FREEDOM: OUR RIGHT TO DECIDE, Marlene Fried & Loretta Ross *(Open Magazine Pamphlet Series*, Pamphlet 18, April, 1992. Main office: P.O. Box 2726, Westfield, N.J., 07091; Europe: Postbus 2126, 1000 CC Amsterdam, Holland. A thoughtful overview of issues involved in the struggle for abortion rights.

THEY WEEP ON MY DOORSTEP, Dr. Ruth Barnett and Doug Baker (Halo Publishers, 1969). P.O. Box 1383, Silver Springs, FL 32688-1383, $7.45. The personal reminiscences of an intrepid naturopath who performed illegal abortions in Portland, Oregon, for 40 years. This book provides an excellent view of the active abortion underground on the West Coast from World War I to the mid-1960s.

UNSURE ABOUT YOUR PREGNANCY? A GUIDE TO MAKING THE RIGHT DECISION FOR YOU, Terry Beresford (1990). Available from the National Abortion Federation, 1436 U St., N.W., #103, Washington, D.C. 20009, (800) 772-9100. Single copies $.50, or quantity discount.

WOMEN & ABORTION: THE BODY AS BATTLEGROUND, Rosayn Baxandall (Open Magazine Pamphlet Series, Pamphlet 17, April 1992. Main office: P.O. Box 2726, Westfield, N.J., 07091; Europe: Postbus 2126, 1000 CC Amsterdam, Holland. Pamphlet 17, April, 1992). This pamphlet provides a brief survey of radical activism that helped pave the way for abortion reform.

PARENTAL NOTIFICATION
AND JUDICIAL BYPASS

NO WAY OUT: YOUNG, PREGNANT AND TRAPPED BY THE LAW American Civil Liberties Union (ACLU) Reproductive Freedom Project, 132 W. 43rd St., New York, NY 10036. This pamphlet contains compelling stories of young women who are confronted with the dilemmas posed by parental notification laws.

PARENTAL NOTICE LAWS: THEIR CATASTROPHIC IMPACT ON TEENAGERS' RIGHT TO ABORTION, The American Civil Liberties Union (ACLU) Reproductive Freedom Project, 1986. A critical, comprehensive indictment of the concept of parental notification and judicial bypass, focusing on the *Hodgson v. Minnesota* case, 1986. (See address above.)

SHATTERING THE DREAMS OF YOUNG WOMEN: THE TRAGIC CONSEQUENCES OF PARENTAL INVOLVEMENT LAWS, American Civil Liberties Union (ACLU) Reproductive Freedom Project, 1991. A brief summary of parental notification laws and their negative impact on young women's lives. (See address above.)

BOOKS ON HERBS

CONTRACEPTION AND ABORTION FROM THE ANCIENT WORLD TO THE RENAISSANCE, John Riddle (Cambridge, MA: Harvard University Press, 1992). This remarkable survey delves into the "hidden" history of fertility control, suggesting that women in ancient time may have possessed knowledge of herbal contraceptives, emmenogues, and abortifacients that modern science has yet to discover.

THE HERB BOOK, John Lust (New York: Bantam Books, 1974). This standard handbook provides a comprehensive overview of herbs used in North America.

SELF-RITUAL FOR INVOKING RELEASE OF SPIRIT LIFE IN THE WOMB: A PERSONAL TREATISE ON RITUAL HERBAL ABORTION, Deborah Maia (Mother Spirit Publishing, P.O. Box 893, Great Barrington, MA, $5.95 + $1.50 p/h.)

WISE WOMAN HERBAL, Susan Weed (Woodstock, NY: Ash Tree Press, 1986). This book has a section on herbal contraceptives and abortifacients.

RU-486

THE ABORTION PILL: RU-486, A WOMAN'S CHOICE, Etienne-Emile Baulieu with Mort Rosenblum (New York: Simon & Schuster, 1991). A lucid, intensely personal account of the development of RU-486 written by the French physician-scientist who spearheaded discovery of the drug, and who has been at the eye of the storm surrounding its marketing.

RU-486: THE PILL THAT COULD END THE ABORTION WARS AND WHY WOMEN DON'T HAVE IT, Lawrence Lader (Reading, MA: Addison-Wesley Publishers, Inc., 1991). This cogent, well-researched book details the development of RU-486, noting briefly the role of Hoechst, A.G., in blocking distribution, but blaming Roussel-Uclaf, the pill's French manufacturer, for refusing to distribute it outside of northern Europe.

VIDEOS ON ABORTION RIGHTS

ABORTION DENIED: SHATTERING YOUNG WOMEN'S LIVES, The Fund for the Feminist Majority, 1600 Wilson Blvd., #704, Arlington, VA 22209 ($29.95). Focused on the story of Becky Bell, this video takes a look at parental consent and notification laws, providing a wealth of hard-hitting facts about the harm these laws cause to young women.

ABORTION FOR SURVIVAL, THE FUND FOR THE FEMINIST MAJORITY ($29.95). This fact-filled video takes a look at the impact of abortion restrictions on women's lives in the U.S., as well as the negative global impact of U.S. government policy on population growth. (See address above.)

ACCESS DENIED, Julie Clark. ReproVision, P.O. Box 2026, New York NY 10009. With the searing immedicy of battlefield footage, this video documents the struggle to defend clinics against the attacks of anti-abortion zealots. The eerie flashbacks to the 1950s remind us of a time when women had little reproductive control, and suggest that if *Roe v. Wade* is overturned or further weakened, menstrual extraction and other non-clinic abortion techniques may offer realistic alternatives to the vagaries of back-alley abortionists.

NO GOING BACK: A PRO-CHOICE PERSPECTIVE, Federation of Feminist Women's Health Centers, 1080 N. Vine St., Los Angeles, CA 90028, #1105 ($29.95). This video contains historic footage of menstrual extraction and includes interviews with Lorraine Rothman, inventor of the Del-EM™, Frank Susman, Chief Counsel for Medical Providers in *Webster v. Reproductive Health Services*; and B.J. Isaacson-Jones, former executive Director of Reproductive Health Services, the clinic named in the *Webster* case.

WITH A VENGEANCE: THE FIGHT FOR REPRODUCTIVE FREEDOM, 1989 (rental $75, sale $600, video $225, available from Women Make Movies, 225 Lafayette St., #207, New York, NY 10012.) This urgent and timely film is a history of the struggle for reproductive freedom since the 1960s, reflecting the wider history of the contemporary women's movement. Rare archival footage and interviews with early abortion rights activists, including members of Red Stockings, Jane, Flo Kennedy and Byllye Avery, are intercut with interviews with young women who testify to the need for multi-racial grassroots coalitions.

NEWSPAPERS/NEWSLETTERS

THE 80% MAJORITY CAMPAIGN, P.O. Box 1315, Hightstown, NJ 08520 (609) 443-8780. Ann Baker, founder of the Campaign, monitors the activities of the anti-abortion movement and keeps the prochoice movement and the media informed of legislative moves, political strategies, demonstrations, pickets, criminal activities, court cases, etc. Baker's periodic newsletter offers a rare inside look at the anti-abortion movement and makes fascinating, if chilling reading.

NEW DIRECTIONS FOR WOMEN, the only national women's newspaper, published bi-monthly, covering a range of women's issues including health, politics, the arts, books, entertainment, women's history, a national calendar of women's events and more. Subscriptions: one year/$12, two years/$20, P.O. Box 3000, Denville, NJ 07834-3000, (800) 562-1973.

SANTA FE HEALTH EDUCATION PROJECT HEALTH LETTER. This monthly health letter provides excellent information on reproductive health issues from an alternative perspective, in English and Spanish. Back issues are available. Order from Santa Fe Health Education Project, P.O. Box 577, Santa Fe, New Mexico, 87504-0577 (505) 982-3236.

WOMENWISE. Now in its 14th year, this quarterly publication of the New Hampshire Feminist Health Centers, includes information and analysis on women's health issues. Available from the New Hampshire Feminist Health Center, 38 S. Main St., Concord, NH 03301 (603) 225-2739 $10 per year.

Index

Rebecca Chalker and **Carol Downer** have been active leaders in the women's health movement for the past 20 years. Rebecca Chalker is the author of *The Complete Cervical Cap Guide* and *Overcoming Bladder Disorders*, named one of the best popular medical books of 1990 by *Library Journal*. Rebecca also co-edited *A New View of a Woman's Body* and *How to Stay Out of the Gynecologist's Office*. She has been an abortion counselor and an active speaker internationally on women's issues. Carol Downer has become a legendary figure in the women's health movement. *Ms.* magazine's poster highlighting 20 years of the U.S. women's movement starts off with Carol's celebrated 1972 trial and acquittal after being charged with practicing medicine without a license for applying yogurt to a vaginal yeast infection. In the early 70's she pioneered the concept of vaginal and cervical self-examination as a key to self-empowerment. A lawyer, she is the founding Executive Director of The Federation of Feminist Women's Health Centers.